Ergonomics for Therapists

Ergonomics For Therapists

Edited by

Karen Jacobs, Ed.D., OTR/L, CPE, FAOTA
Clinical Assistant Professor of Occupational Therapy
Boston University
Boston, Massachusetts

Carl M. Bettencourt, OTR/L
Biomechanics Specialist
The Hillhaven Corporation/Blueberry Hill Healthcare
Beverly, Massachusetts

Butterworth–Heinemann
Boston London Oxford Singapore Sydney Toronto Wellington

Library of Congress Cataloging-in-Publication Data

Ergonomics for therapists / edited by Karen Jacobs, Carl M. Bettencourt.
     p.   cm.
  Includes bibliographical references and index.
  ISBN 0-7506-9530-7
  1. Occupational therapy. 2. Human engineering. 3. Physical
therapy. I. Jacobs, Karen, 1951- . II. Bettencourt, Carl M.
  [DNLM: 1. Disabled—rehabilitation. 2. Human Engineering.
3. Occupational Therapy. 4. Occupational Health. WB 320 E665
1994]
  RM735.E73 1994
  615.8'515—dc20
  DNLM/DLC
  for Library of Congress   94-35496
                                        CIP

British Library Cataloguing-in-Publication Data
A catalogue record for this book is available from the British Library.

Butterworth-Heinemann
313 Washington Street
Newton, MA 02158

10 9 8 7 6 5 4 3 2 1

Printed in the United States of America

Contents

IV. The Application Process

Appendixes

Preface

Ergonomic consultation is a growing service provided by occupational and physical therapists who have advanced knowledge and skills in this area. *Ergonomics for Therapists* has been designed as a reference for therapists who are interested in acquiring knowledge, tools, and techniques in ergonomics. This text is not a substitute for continuing education and advanced academic training in ergonomics and related fields but is a complement to lifelong learning.

To provide a framework for understanding ergonomics, the text has been divided into four parts. Part I provides a general overview of ergonomics; Part II defines and describes some of the knowledge, tools, and techniques that ergonomics encompasses; Part III discusses topics of special consideration; and Part IV applies ergonomics to occupational and physical therapy practice.

To begin a book takes an act of will, but to complete it requires the assistance and support of many. Appreciation is due everyone who helped in the journey. Most important, we thank the contributing authors, who eagerly shared their expertise and insights. Deep gratitude is extended to research assistants: Sara Hill, Erin Dunkerley, and Lorraine Vaccaro. We gratefully thank the editorial staff at Butterworth-Heinemann for their assistance, in particular Associate Editor, Medical Books, Karen Oberheim. Much appreciation is extended to Niels Buessem for his encouragement in the writing of this book. Finally, we thank our families and friends for their continued support.

K.J.
C.M.B.

Contributing Authors

Diane Aja, M.S., OTR
Outpatient Service Coordinator, Department of Occupational Therapy, Work Enhancement and Rehabilitation Center, Medical Center Hospital of Vermont, Colchester
    Chapter 8: Revised 1991 NIOSH Equation for the Design and Evaluation of Manual Lifting Tasks

Joe Barry, M.S., OTR/L
Staff Occupational Therapist, Department of Occupational Therapy, New England Rehabilitation Hospital, Woburn, Massachusetts
    Chapter 10: Keyboards

Carl M. Bettencourt, OTR/L
Biomechanics Specialist, The Hillhaven Corporation/Blueberry Hill Healthcare, Beverly, Massachusetts
    Chapter 11: Ergonomics and Injury Prevention Programs

Joann Marie Brooks, M.P.H., P.T., O.C.S.
Adjunct Faculty, Department of Physical Therapy, Massachusetts General Hospital Institute of Health Professions, Boston; Outpatient Rehabilitation Services Manager, Department of Physical and Occupational Therapy, Columbia/HCA Portsmouth Regional Hospital, Portsmouth, New Hampshire
    Chapter 7: Lifting Testing and Analysis

David J. Folts, OTR/L
Work Hardening Coordinator, Physical Therapy Department, Warren Occupational Rehabilitation Center, Warren, Ohio
    Chapter 4: Cognitive Workload

A. James Giannini, M.D.
Professor of Psychiatry, Ohio State University, Columbus; Medical Director, Chemical Abuse Centers, Inc., Austintown, Ohio
    Chapter 4: Cognitive Workload

Diane C. Hermenau, M.S., OTR/L
Clinical Supervisor, Department of Occupational Therapy, Morton Hospital and Medical Center, Taunton, Massachusetts
        Chapter 9: Seating

Karen Jacobs, Ed.D., OTR/L, CPE, FAOTA
Clinical Assistant Professor of Occupational Therapy, Boston University, Boston; editor of *Work: A Journal of Prevention, Assessment, and Rehabilitation*
        Chapter 12: Marketing Ergonomic Consultation; 13: Certification in Ergonomics

Bonnie Lynne Otonicar, OTR/L
Manager, Industrial Rehabilitation and Contract Services, Return to Work Department, Lorain Community Hospital, Lorain, Ohio
        Chapter 4: Cognitive Workload

Peter Picone, M.S.I.E.
Staff Ergonomist and Engineering Systems Analyst, Department of Logistics, Dynamic Research Corporation (DRC), Wilmington, Massachusetts
        Chapter 5: Environmental Design

Lt. Col. Valerie J. Berg Rice, Ph.D., OTR/L, CPE
Research Occupational Therapist, Occupational Physiology Division, Occupational Health and Performance Directorate, U.S. Army Research Institute of Environmental Medicine, Natick, Massachusetts
        Chapter 1: Ergonomics: An Introduction; 6: Human Factors in Medical Rehabilitation Equipment: Product Development and Usability Testing

Robin Chandler Sutherland, OTR/L
Executive Director, New England Spine Care Center, Chestnut Hill, Massachusetts
        Chapter 2: Anthropometry

Laurie A. Vincello, M.A., P.T.
Physical Therapy Supervisor, The New England Spine Care Center, Chestnut Hill, Massachusetts
        Chapter 3: Basic Biomechanics

PART I

Overview

CHAPTER 1

Ergonomics: An Introduction

Valerie J. Berg Rice

ABSTRACT

Ergonomics is defined, and a brief history of the field of ergonomics is provided. The interrelationship between therapists and ergonomists in the following three areas of practice is described: (1) work-site analysis, (2) environmental and product design for populations with physical challenges, and (3) research.

The musculoskeletal ergonomic concepts that underlie injury prevention and safety are not new to therapists. The origin of an injury is typically noted during a therapist's initial evaluation of a client. When a trend is noted over several work-related incidents, therapists develop educational and preventive strategies and provide consultation in the work setting to eliminate or reduce identifiable problems. Therapists explain the mechanism of an injury to their clients as a precaution against additional damage or exacerbation of the symptoms. For example, clients with back injuries are taught proper methods of lifting and carrying, and they are instructed in the theories of injury and wellness related to their condition. The same is true for all categories of illness and injury. Educational and preventive strategies are thus introduced into the workplace on the basis of client reports.

In the field of occupational therapy, the fundamental goal is "the capacity [of the client or patient] throughout the life span, to perform with satisfaction to self and others those tasks and roles essential to productive living and to the mastery of self and the environment" (Hopkins, 1978, p. 27).

Although the wording may be unfamiliar to those who are not occupational therapists, the goal is understood: to assist clients in attaining their highest functional performance in all areas of life, including work, recreation, and home. To treat clients so that they are able to return to their work roles, therapists must be aware of clients' limitations and capabilities in their current state, their potential abilities, and the physiologic and psychologic demands of their work. In addition, therapists must be aware of the performance competencies and confines of people without injuries to be able to assess whether or not a client is functioning within normal range. Maximal functional performance has been the goal of occupational therapy since the inception of the profession in 1917 (beginning with the founding of the National Society for the Promotion of Occupational Therapy). The use of purposeful activity, such as work tasks and work simulation, as treatment modalities was integral to the development of the profession and is identified in the name of the profession, *occupational* therapy.

Early in the development of the field of physical therapy, the fundamental intent was "to assess, prevent, and treat movement dysfunction and physical disability, with the overall goal of enhancing human movement and function" (McMillan, as cited by Pinkston, 1989, p. 2). These goals conform to the intentions delineated by ergonomists and human factors engineers, especially those who design workplaces and equipment with physical safety and effective work performance in mind. For example, as industrial consultants, physical therapists use their knowledge of human motion to evaluate safe and effective working postures. Physical therapists who work in an industrial environment also evaluate injured workers' limitations and capabilities (functional capacity assessment) and the demands of the work role (job-site analysis) to establish treatment regimens. Assessment and treatment roles may be targeted toward specialty areas, such as back care, strength training, or work hardening (use of job simulation in treatment). The benefits of having an occupational therapist or physical therapist on the ergonomic team are the increased likelihood of early return to work of injured employees, matching worker capabilities with work demands, and the prevention of injuries. Each of these benefits can translate into increased revenues for a company (Key, 1989).

Good principles of ergonomics are most noted when they are absent, since their focus is to optimize the relationship between the environment and the person (Kantowitz & Sorkin, 1983). When an appropriate ergonomic design is in use, the user should be unaware of environmental design deficiencies and be able to concentrate on the task at hand. For example, in a well-designed office workstation, a worker should not have to hold his or her neck in an awkward posture to use a visual display terminal (VDT) and should not experience neck and shoulder discomfort. According to Osborne (1982), good ergonomic design in the workplace offers a means to "victory over the oppressive forces which continue to make work less productive, less pleasant, less comfortable and less safe."

In the past, industry focused on work demands while the needs of workers took second place. Humanistic and economic concerns and litigation, however, have convinced industry that consideration of the worker is good business. The use of sound ergonomic principles has generated many examples of increased worker productivity and safety. One example (Chaney & Teel, 1967) demonstrated that less training is required if workers' abilities are considered in the design of equipment. In this example, the detection efficiency of machine parts inspectors was evaluated after either a 4-hour training program or use of a set of visual aids and displays that assisted with the detection of defects. A 32% increase in detected defects was found with the training, a 42% increase was found with the use of appropriate visual aids, and a 71% increase was found when training and visual aids were combined. Although training was useful, a properly designed environment would also be needed for superior results.

Ergonomics Defined

Ergonomics (Greek *ergon* "work" + Greek *nomos* "law") focuses on the study of work performance with an emphasis on worker safety and productivity. Several definitions have been proposed. One of the best definitions of ergonomics was provided by Chapanis (1991), who used the terms *ergonomics* and *human factors* synonymously. He wrote, "Human factors (ergonomics) is a body of knowledge about human abilities, human limitations, and other human characteristics that are relevant to design. *Human factors engineering* (ergonomics implementation) is the application of human factors information to the design of tools, machines, systems, tasks, jobs, and environments for safe, comfortable, and effective human use" (Chapanis, 1991, p. 2).

There has been considerable debate on the definitions of *ergonomics* and *human factors*. The controversy has been especially fervent regarding the differentiation as opposed to the interchangeability of the terms. The proponents of differentiating the terms argue that the term *human factors* was first used in psychology, whereas *ergonomics* originated in human physiology and biomechanics (Fraser, 1989). The differentiation is capricious at best, and the major human factors and ergonomics texts encourage the use of the two terms interchangeably (Gay, 1986; Fraser, 1989; Meister, 1989; Wilson & Corlett, 1990). In their introductory text, Sanders and McCormick (1987, p. 4) state that "some people have tried to distinguish between the two, but we believe that any distinctions are arbitrary and that, for all practical purposes, the terms are synonymous."

In this chapter, as well as throughout the entire book, the two terms are used interchangeably. It is true that *ergonomics* has not been as widely used in the United States and Canada as in other parts of the world. In the United States, the terms *human factors engineering, human engineering, engineering psychology,* and *human factors* have been used. The current favorite is *human factors*. As noted by Chapanis (1991, p. 2), "whether we call ourselves human factors engineers or ergonomists is mostly an accident of where we happen to live and where we were trained." *Ergonomics* is quickly becoming the more recognized term among the general public, even in the United States.

Ergonomics focuses on humans and their interactions with the environment. It involves interactions with tools, equipment, consumer products, work methods, jobs, instruction books, facilities, and organizations. As noted by Kantowitz and Sorkin (1983, p. 13), "the first commandment of human factors is 'Honor Thy User'." Ergonomists design environments and products according to the physical (visual, auditory, tactile, strength, anthropometric), cognitive (learning, information-processing, retention), and psychologic (cultural influences, behavior, background) characteristics of humans. Accordingly, ergonomics is not solely confined to the workplace. Products and environments should match the abilities, needs, and perceptions of the people who use and exist in them. In self care, there are ergonomically designed toothbrushes and spigots. These spigots conform to users expectations, that is, that water should emerge when the spigot is turned counterclockwise and that cold water should be controlled by the spigot on the user's right. Bicycles and snow skis are designed with riders and skiers of differing abilities in mind and are designed differently for men and women. There are numerous examples in homes and offices of proper and improper ergonomic designs. It is clear that the concept of making the devices and systems "user friendly" extends beyond the workplace.

To attain the goal of designing user-friendly devices and systems, ergonomists conduct scientific investigations to identify the limitations, capabilities, and responses of humans in a variety of climates and circumstances. This information is then used to produce designs that match human characteristics. The first part of this book, "Knowledge, Tools, and Techniques," provides examples of how physical and cognitive information can be applied in the workplace. The second part, "Special Considerations," demonstrates how human characteristics are applied to specific situations. Ergonomists evaluate equipment, jobs, work methods, and environments to ensure they meet their intended objectives. The chapter on usability testing describes the procedures for conducting an ergonomic evaluation of rehabilitation equipment.

Ergonomics can be considered a design philosophy that focuses on producing a design that ensures safety, ease of use, comfort, and efficiency. However, many distinguished human factors practitioners/ergonomists believe that human factors/ergonomics is a unitary, scholarly discipline with unique characteristics, just as occupational therapy and physical therapy are unique disciplines (Meister, 1989).

History of Ergonomics

Although the concept of human factors/ergonomics existed during the stone age (as humans constructed tools to fit their own hands and hunting and gathering needs), the field of study began as technologic developments were made during the industrial revolution. Time and motion studies are considered predecessors of human factors/ergonomics. Time and motion studies focused on evaluation of work methods, workstation design, and equipment design. They were conducted by numerous investigators, including the Gilbreths, Taylor, Muensterberg, and Binet (Christensen, 1987).

The field of ergonomics received particular attention during World War II, when the complexity of military equipment surpassed the abilities of the human operators (Damon & Randall, 1944). "Man had become the weak link" (Damon et al, 1966, p. 2). As during World War I, the primary focus was selection and training of personnel; however, even with extensive training, the personnel could not always perform as needed (Sanders & McCormick, 1987). Because humans cannot be redesigned and because selection and training were not providing an acceptable solution, the focus changed to fitting the task to the person by using human dimensions, capabilities, and limitations in the design process.

After World War II, the Ergonomics Research Society (the current Ergonomics Society) was founded in England, and the first ergonomics and human factors text, *Applied Experimental Psychology: Human Factors in Engineering Design* by Chapanis, Garner, and Morgan, was published (1949). In 1957, the Human Factors Society was formed in the United States, and the journal *Ergonomics*, the journal of the Ergonomics Research Society, began publication. The International Ergonomics Association was formed in 1959 to join ergonomics and human factors societies from several countries. Since that time the field of ergonomics has experienced tremendous growth and the development of areas of specialization. Computer technology introduced the specialization in the interface between humans and computers, and the incident at Three-Mile Island accelerated the role of human factors and ergonomics in the nuclear power industry. In addition, product liability increased the number of human factors/ergonomics experts needed in forensics to address design deficiencies, instructions, and warning labels (Sanders & McCormick, 1987).

Ergonomics developed from the common interests of a number of professions, particularly engineering, psychology, and medicine. It has remained a multidisciplinary field of study. Present-day ergonomists include professionals with degrees in psychology, engineering, human factors/ergonomics, industrial design, education, physiology, medicine, allied health, business administration, computer science, and industrial hygiene.

The Interrelationship Between Therapists and Ergonomists

The interrelationship between rehabilitation and ergonomics has received a great deal of attention (Rice, 1992). Therapists and ergonomists share common interests, and therapists can contribute to the practice of ergonomics in three major areas in addition to integrating ergonomic principles into therapeutic clinical practice. These areas are worksite analysis aimed at prevention of cumulative musculoskeletal trauma; workplace and tool design for individuals with disabilities; and the development and use of databases. In addition, there is some crossover in the research interests of rehabilitation professionals and human factors engineers and ergonomists.

Worksite Analysis

It is important for therapists to be familiar with the field of ergonomics as a whole, so that they understand the language being used, know how to best describe their own expertise, and recognize when an ergonomist with specialized training should be consulted. A review of introductory ergonomics texts produced the following observations about the knowledge base of therapists compared with ergonomists (Kantowitz & Sorkin, 1983; Osborne, 1982; Sanders & McCormick, 1987).

Some areas of ergonomics with which therapists are familiar are the sensory nervous system, anthropometry, kinesiology, human development, anatomy and physiology, work capability analysis, and basic research. Areas that are familiar to occupational therapists (and to physical therapists, depending on their training) include communication, learning, motivation, and normal and abnormal psychology (including the effects of stress), job and task analysis, and measures of job satisfaction. Workplace design, seating and posture, and safety may or may not be included in the knowledge of entry-level therapists. Topics in ergonomics with which entry-level therapists may be unfamiliar include person-machine communication (displays and controls), workstation design, vibration, noise, temperature, illumination, training, inspection and maintenance, error and reliability, signal detection theory, visual displays, legal aspects of product liability, and advanced statistical research.

Therapists are well educated in the procedures of problem identification, interviewing, observation, and record review. Their considerable knowledge in anatomy and physiology, neuroanatomy and neurophysiology, kinesiology, anthropometry, and the mechanism and treatment of injuries makes therapists considerable allies for ergonomists. Knowledge of ergonomics allows therapists to apply their expertise by specializing in the field of musculoskeletal ergonomics and safety.

The application of ergonomics for therapists primarily implies worksite consultation directed at preventing musculoskeletal injuries. The goals are to promote safety and to decrease the financial costs associated with lost work time, medical treatment, and retraining. Consultative services can be combined with direct services (client treatment) or can be offered alone. When providing consultative services in addition to direct services, a therapist can offer functional capacity testing, work hardening, and graded return-to-work placements along with work-site evaluations. Ergonomic work-site evaluations may include task analysis, videotaping, measurement and analysis of equipment and workstation, and workspace analysis. The last part of this book addresses the ergonomic intervention process from the beginning (program development and marketing) through problem identification, analysis, and implementation to the final product (evaluation and report of results).

Design for Individuals with Disabilities

More than 43 million Americans have physical or mental disabilities. According to the Committee on a National Agenda for the Prevention of Disabilities, one in seven Americans has a disabling condition (Bello, 1991; Pope & Tarlov, 1991). Cannon, a human factors consultant in Colorado who has designed equipment for the visually impaired, stated, "No segment of the population suffers more from neglect of human factors requirements in product design than the severely handicapped" (Gay, 1986, p. 99). Many factors contribute to this lapse, but the need for a database, the expense of small projects, and the lack of knowledge regarding usability testing can be alleviated by proper ergonomic consideration.

Few data exist on the anthropometric characteristics, capabilities, and limitations of individuals with disabilities and elderly populations in varying climates and conditions. The argument that has prevented the collection of such information is that the capabilities and limitations differ with each disease process and with each person. This argument could also be made for the able-bodied population. Capabilities and limitations differ according to one's genetic background and training. Individual differences also exist. However, until the abilities and restrictions of individuals with disabilities and elderly populations are identified, suitable products will not be developed on a consistent basis. The expansion of the older population has resulted in an increased interest in geriatrics. Consequently, more geriatric research has been generated. However, a commensurate increase in research for individuals with disabilities has not occurred. The resistance, location, and shape of hand and foot controls; workplace design for people who must sit; and seat pan depth and width requirements differ for people with disabilities and vary according to the disabling condition. Therapists have the skills and are in the setting to gather information for a database on various populations with disabilities.

Technologic aids for individuals with disabilities are expensive because small-scale production is not cost-effective. Although this situation may continue for high-level technologic equipment, it is unknown if assistive equipment would be attractive and useful for the able-bodied population. For example, use of large numerals on telephones; large, well-marked keys on television remote controls; and door levers rather than knobs may be equally desirable for both disabled and able-bodied populations. Only through appropriate usability evaluations will such information become available. Therapists and medical practitioners must become aware of the need for and must develop skills in usability testing. Medical and rehabilitation equipment must be designed with the users (medical practitioners and clients) in mind. Appropriate ergonomic design could increase user acceptance, decrease errors, and increase productivity.

Therapists can provide ergonomists and design engineers with valuable information on the functional capabilities and limitations of, environmental effects on, and overall prognosis of individual clients and of diagnostic groups. The information is essential to identifying needed accommodations, which is particularly important as industry works to implement the Americans with Disabilities Act (ADA).

Research Interests

Therapists and ergonomists often need the same information on human performance. Therapists can and do use ergonomic data in clinical treatment and prevention programs. For example, when treating hospitalized clients, it is important that a therapist be aware of the effects of diurnal variation on muscle strength during muscle strength testing and be aware of the effects of sleep deprivation on cognition, perceptual-motor performance, and learning. Therapists use ergonomic data during the evaluation of, goal setting with, and treatment of clients. The same kinds of information are used by human factors/ergonomics professionals to recommend design improvements for equipment used by able-bodied and individuals with disabilities (Sanders & McCormick, 1987). In addition, therapists contribute to the knowledge of human performance, neurosensory function, and strength testing.

Conclusion

Although a definition of *ergonomics* has been identified, it is important to recognize what ergonomics is not. Ergonomics is not simply "1) applying checklists and guidelines, 2) using oneself as the model for designing objects, or 3) common sense" (Sanders & McCormick, 1987, p. 6). A "cookbook" approach to ergonomics is an embarrassment to the therapist or ergonomist who uses it and is inherently dangerous.

Ergonomics is a satisfying area of specialization for therapists. It provides therapists with a growth area for injury prevention. It also is an area that presents considerable challenge for designing better equipment for the clients therapists serve. Clients deserve to be considered in the design of their equipment and environments. Therapists have the skills, knowledge, and abilities to contribute in the field of ergonomics, and this book provides information and tools to enhance that process.

References

AOTA Fact Sheet (1993). Questions and answers: Careers in occupational therapy. Rockville, Md.: American Occupational Therapy Association.

Bello, M. (1991). Preventing disability demands new thinking: Looking toward a national agenda. News Report, XLI, 3:2-4.

Chaney, F.B., Teel, K.S. (1967). Improving inspector performance through training and visual aids. Journal of Applied Psychology, 51:311-315.

Chapanis, A. (1991). To communicate the human factors message, you have to know what the message is and how to communicate it. Human Factors Society Bulletin, 34: 1-4.

Chapanis, A., Garner, W.R., and Morgan, C.T. (1949). Applied Experimental Psychology. New York: Wiley.

Christensen, J.M. (1987). The human factors profession. In G. Salvendy (Ed.), Handbook of Human Factors (pp. 4-15). New York: Wiley.

Damon, A., Randall F.E. (1944). Physical anthropology in the Army Air Forces. American Journal of Physical Anthropology, 2:293-316.

Damon, A., Stoudt, H.W., McFarland, R.A. (1966). The Human Body in Equipment Design. Cambridge, Mass.: Harvard University Press.

Fraser, T.M. (1989). The Worker at Work: A Textbook Concerned with Men and Women in the Workplace. New York: Taylor & Francis.

Gay, K. (1986). Ergonomics: Making Products and Places Fit People. Hillside, N.J.: Enslow.

Hopkins, H.L. (1978). Current basis for theory and philosophy of occupational therapy. In Willard and Spackman, Occupational Theory. Philadelphia: Lippincott.

Kantowitz, B.H., and Sorkin, R.D. (1983). Human Factors: Understanding People-System Relationships. New York: Wiley.

Key, G.L. (1989). Work Capacity Analysis. In R.M. Scully and M.R. Barnes (Eds.), Physical Therapy. New York: Lippincott.

Meister, D. (1989). Conceptual Aspects of Human Factors. Baltimore: Johns Hopkins University Press.

Occupational Therapy: Its Definition and Function (1972). American Journal of Occupational Therapy, 26:204.

Osborne, D.J. (1982). Ergonomics at Work. New York: Wiley.

Pinkston, D. (1989). Evolution of the Practice of Physical Therapy in the United States. In R.M. Scully and M.R. Barnes (Eds.), Physical Therapy. New York: Lippincott.

Pope, A.M., Tarlov, A.R. (Eds.) (1991). Committee on a National Agenda for the Prevention of Disabilities, Division of Health Promotion and Disease Prevention, National Institute of Medicine. Washington, D.C.: National Academy Press.

Rice, V.J. (1992). Defining common ground: human factors engineering and rehabilitation. Rehab Management, 5:30-32.

Sanders, M.S., and McCormick, E.J. (1987). Human Factors in Engineering and Design. New York: McGraw-Hill.

Smith, K.U. (1987). Origins of human factors science. Human Factors Society Bulletin, 30:1-3.

Wilson, J.R., and Corlett, E.N. (Eds.) (1990). Evaluation of Human Work: A Practical Ergonomics Methodology. New York: Taylor & Francis.

PART II

Knowledge, Tools, and Techniques

CHAPTER 2

Anthropometry

Robin Chandler Sutherland

ABSTRACT

Anthropometry is fundamental to ergonomic practice.
Anthropometric principles and data are intertwined
with ergonomics in the design of workstations, furniture, equipment, and tools. It is not enough to design a
workplace to suit the average worker; anthropometric
analysis promotes optimal function and safety for a targeted population. Therapists must be able to apply anthropometric data to the workplace to optimize job
performance, minimize fatigue, and prevent cumulative
musculoskeletal trauma. This chapter acquaints therapists with the basic principles of anthropometry and
their application to the workstation.

Anthropometry is central to designing facilities, equipment, furniture, tools,
and personal protective devices. Anthropometric data are a collection of
measurements of large numbers of humans that are used to establish average
size ranges. Once measurements such as height, reach, hip width, and hand
size are known, the design of workstations and work becomes scientific,
allowing the greatest percentage of the working force to be within safe limits
in the design of work and workspaces.

Because many of the early anthropometric data were collected from
studies of the military, the resulting designs for the most part accommodated
young men. Because the work force has changed, including an increase in the

15

number of female and older workers, anthropometric data have expanded to include all categories of working people. The correlation of anthropometric norms with actual work forces is crucial—individualized data (eg, height, weight, age, strength, sex) about a work force allow appropriate anthropometric data to be selected. Companies that perform anthropometric studies on their own work force have the most accurate data and thus have the necessary information to design ergonomically sound workstations.

Natural postures are attitudes of the trunk and extremities that do not involve static effort. Natural postures and movements are a necessary part of efficient work; therefore, it is essential that the workplace be suited to the body size of the operator. Because there are enormous variations in body size among individuals, the two sexes, and the different races, it is not enough to design a workplace to suit the average worker. It is necessary to consider the body dimensions of all workers who may be placed at a given workstation.

Awkward postures during work tasks may be a result of several factors, including poor workstation design, the design attributes of tools and equipment, incorrect work methods, and poor body mechanics. Posture may be affected by the anthropometric attributes of a worker relative to the location and orientation of the workstation. If not relieved, awkward postures can cause localized muscle fatigue, mechanical stress on the intervertebral disks, back pain and disability, and other musculoskeletal disorders. Awkward postures are of particular concern for workers who perform highly repetitive jobs because of the frequency and cumulative effects of exposure (Carlett & Bishop, 1976; Grandjean, 1980; National Institute for Occupational Health and Safety [NIOSH], 1981).

Standing Work

An intervertebral disk is a cushion that separates two vertebrae. A disk consists of viscous fluid enclosed in tough fibrous rings. These disks collectively give flexibility to the spine. Over time the disks degenerate and lose their strength. The degenerative process impairs the mechanics of the vertebral column and allows tissues and nerves to be strained and pinched, leading to back pain. Unnatural postures, lifting heavy weights, and prolonged poor sitting postures can accelerate the deterioration of the disks.

Research conducted at the University of Michigan on spinal compression forces for selected trunk postures (Chaffin & Andersson, 1984; Keyserling et al, 1987) demonstrated that nonneutral trunk postures can produce biomechanical stresses that approach the safety limits for spinal disk compression forces established by NIOSH. For example, trunk flexion of 10 degrees produces a compression force of 783 newtons (N), but this force increases to 1207 N at 20 degrees of flexion, 1939 N at 45 degrees of flexion, and 2278 N at 90 degrees. For a job to be considered "acceptable" by NIOSH, spinal compression forces cannot exceed 3430 N (NIOSH, 1981). A person who holds his or her trunk in 45 degrees of flexion while carrying no weight in his or her hands already exceeds 50 percent of the threshold for acceptability specified by NIOSH.

In a review of the effect of awkward working postures, trunk flexion was associated with reports of transient local muscle fatigue and back pain (Dullis & Contini, 1985). Nonneutral postures have been demonstrated to increase considerably the biochemical strain induced in the lower back, such as the forces exerted by the erector spinae muscles, intradiskal pressure, and compression forces on the spinal disks (Andersson et al, 1977; Chaffin, 1973; Van Wely, 1970).

Head and neck postures are difficult to assess because seven joints determine the mobility of this part of the body. For example, it is possible to combine an erect or extended (lordotic) neck with a flexed, downward bent head or a flexed (kyphotic) neck with an upward directed head.

Because ergonomic recommendations for the dimensions of workstations are based on anthropometric data only to some extent, behavioral patterns of employees and specific requirements of the work itself must be considered. Thus, the recommended dimensions given in textbooks are generally compromise solutions, which can be quite arbitrary and should not be used independently of the other considerations. For example, working heights are critical in the design of workstations. If a station is too high for a worker, the worker must lift his or her shoulders to compensate for the lack of height in relation to the station, resulting in painful cramps in the neck and shoulders. If a station is too low, the worker's back may be bowed for extended periods of time, resulting in a backache.

Anthropometric studies of the United States civilian population show an average height of 177 cm (69 inches) for men and 161.5 cm (63.5 inches) for women (National Aeronautics and Space Administration [NASA], 1978). The corresponding shoulder height is 145 cm (57 inches) for the average man and 132 cm (52 inches) for the average woman (Dullis & Contini, 1985). The amount of shoulder flexion required during a task is inversely related to the operator's height. For example, a short person may be required to flex the shoulder more than a tall person during a machine operation task. The most favorable work height for handwork when standing is 50 to 100 mm below the elbow.

In addition to anthropometric measurements, the nature of the work must be considered. For delicate (fine motor) work, supporting the elbows reduces the static loads on the muscles of the back; a good work height is generally 50 to 100 mm above the elbow. During manual work, in which space is often needed for equipment, tools, and materials, a suitable height is 100 to 150 mm below the elbow. If considerable effort must be exerted by the upper body (eg, heavy assembly work), the work surface should be 150 to 400 mm below elbow height (Grandjean, 1988).

Thus, ergonomically it is desirable to be able to adjust the working heights of stations to suit individual workers. If for financial or practical reasons a firm is unable to provide fully adjustable benches, or if the operating level at a workstation cannot be varied, then the work height should be set to suit the tallest operator. The taller person thus avoids excessive trunk flexion, and the shorter operators can be accommodated with a platform on which to stand.

Reaching

Lifting the shoulders is strenuous static work. Workers often compensate for a working level that is too high by lifting their shoulders through contraction of the trapezius muscle or lifting the upper arms with the deltoid muscle. The contraction force of these muscles over a period of time generates great pain in the shoulder region. Prolonged elevation of the arms (shoulder flexion or abduction) causes extreme muscle fatigue and, in some cases, acute tendinitis (Keyserling, 1986a). Shoulder abduction and extension have been cited as postural stresses related to the development of thoracic outlet syndrome (Keyserling, 1986b). Neutral positions of the shoulder are considered to be flexion and abduction below a 45-degree angle.

Understanding how much room the hands and arms need to grasp objects and move them about is an important factor in the planning of controls, tools, accessories, and work surfaces. Reaching too far for items leads to excessive trunk movement, making the operation itself less accurate and less efficient than it would be under ideal ergonomic conditions and increasing the risk for pain in the back and shoulders.

Vertical grasp is the radius of arm movement with the hands in a grasping position. The vertical grasp in the sagittal plane of the body is an arc of radius 610 mm above shoulder height for men and 550 mm above shoulder height for women (Grandjean, 1988). If lateral movements of the arm are allowed, then the grasping space becomes a semicircular shell of comparable radius (Grandjean, 1988). An occasional stretch to reach beyond this range is permissible because the momentary effect on the trunk and shoulders is minimal.

Trunk flexion of 20 degrees lowers the shoulders and moves them forward, slightly increasing reach limits in the horizontal and vertical planes (Keyserling et al, 1988). This allows a worker a slightly greater reach limit than simply the length of the reach radius. In the construction of workstations, caution must be exercised to minimize the use of maximum reach; repeated reaching to these limits may cause muscle fatigue and soft-tissue injury. In general, repetitive or prolonged reaching should be limited to a distance of about one-half the reach radius, defined as one-half the distance from the shoulder to fingers in a fully extended arm (Keyserling et al, 1988). In other words, workers should not raise their elbows above chest height during repetitive or prolonged reaching (Armstrong, 1987; Bjelle et al, 1979;

Grandjean, 1988); if workers follow this guideline, their arm movement will not exceed 60 degrees of shoulder flexion.

In the development of criteria for establishing workstation reach limits, anthropometric data should be utilized to accommodate 95% of the male and female working populations represented. To do this, the design should simultaneously satisfy the 95th percentile male body-size stereotype and the 5th percentile female body-size stereotype. For example, objects that are close to the body must be positioned within the reach of a large (95th percentile) man, because the low reach limit for a large man is more constrained than the low reach limit of a small woman because of height differences. Another example would be positioning objects within the reach of a small (5th percentile) woman, who has a shorter reach radius than a large man.

Seated Work

During the early 20th century, the idea gradually emerged that work efficiency is improved and fatigue reduced when people sit to do their work. While a person is standing, an outlay of static muscular effort is required to keep the joints of the feet, knees, and hips in fixed positions; this effort ceases when the person sits. This realization led to a greater application of medical and ergonomic concepts to the design of seats for work. This development gained in importance as increasingly more workers sat at their jobs; approximately three-fourths of the work force in industrialized countries now performs work while sitting.

An important disadvantage of sitting is that intervertebral disk pressure is greater than when a person is standing (Nachemson & Morris, 1964). The highest level of disk pressure at 100 kg occurs in unsupported sitting with the spine in a kyphotic position. However, as lumbar support increases, disk pressure decreases; disk pressure is lowest when the lumbar spine is in lordosis. The use of arm rests results in a decrease in disk pressure (Andersson, 1974). Therefore, the disk pressure is at its lowest when low-back support is provided so that a lordotic position is maintained and the weight of the arms is supported.

Many different chairs are on the market because there are many opinions and varying requirements regarding the ideal seat because there are anthropometric data on various populations. Regardless of use, however, it is important to be able to adjust any chair to meet the basic anthropometric dimensions of the worker.

Guiding principles in the selection of seating are as follows:

• The seat surface should be 3 to 5 cm below the fold of the knee when the worker is standing.
• Foot supports should be used with seats that are higher than normal.

- The width of the seat should be sufficient to accommodate the users.
- The depth of the seat should allow the user to rest against the backrest to reduce disk load.
- The backrest must have a well-formed lumbar pad, which should offer good support at a height of 100 to 200 mm above the lowest point of the seat.
- The backrest must be adjustable for the user.

Armrests are an important feature of a chair. They must be evaluated for length, width, height, width between armrests, and the distance from armrest front to seat front. If armrests are too high or if the armrest-to-armrest width is too large, the user must raise the shoulders and abduct the arms. On the other hand, if the armrest is too low, the worker can use it only by sliding forward or leaning to one side. Armrests must be placed so as not to become obstacles; when armrests are too high or too wide, they can prevent the worker from sliding the chair under a work surface. (See Chapter 9 for further discussion.)

Work Surfaces

The height and design of the work surface cannot be the same for all types of work. Three factors determine the type of work surface to be selected: material size, movements demanded to perform a task and the overall work layout. For each type of work, adjustability is advantageous to ensure proper fit to the worker. The qualities of a work surface to be evaluated are top height, bottom height, and slope. The work surface must be large enough to accommodate the objects required for the work. When controls are used, they must be placed within the optimum work area.

The bottom height of the work surface must allow ample leg room. Work heights must be adjustable, however, when force must be exerted during arm and hand work. This need for a low work surface conflicts with the necessity for knee room. A work surface 740 to 780 mm high allows the most range for adaptation, provided that foot rests and an adjustable seat are available (Chaffin, 1973).

The field of vision is of utmost importance to prevent forward flexion of the neck and trunk. A focal distance of 20 to 40 cm is common. The height of a work surface should be related to the position of the elbow. It is important to remember that the work surface height is not always the table height: for example, when a typewriter or computer is being used, the surface height is the keyboard height. Principles determining the height of a work surface are as follows:

- The armrests should be of an appropriate height and length for the user and the desk.

- The back of the chair should be easily reached.
- The lumbar support should be at the correct height or should be adjustable.
- When the user is seated, his or her head should be erect. The line of vision should be horizontal with the first line of characters on a computer screen. The distance should be 500 to 600 mm.
- The user's shoulders should be relaxed and the upper arms should be parallel to the trunk.
- The user's elbows should be flexed at least 90° while the person is working.
- The feet should be fully supported on either the floor or a footstool.
- The work surface should be organized so that all materials, equipment, and controls are within optimum reach, so that the user avoids continual reaching.

If all these factors are considered, an individual user at a workstation should be able to perform the required duties in a manner that promotes productivity and minimizes discomfort. If, however, a workstation is used by several individuals, the original design may not be appropriate. A therapist may have to evaluate each worker from an anthropometric standpoint. If the workstation is identical throughout a large company, for example, 300 workers performing similar work at similar stations, the task for a therapist broadens, and so must the use of available resources. Anthropometric data for a population similar to the work force at the company may then be utilized. If the company employs 300 workers at similar workstations over a large geographic territory, demographic differences may require a different approach from that used if the workers were all in one location. A therapist should understand anthropometric principles and applications so that optimum results are achieved when designing, modifying, or recommending adaptations or equipment for a workspace.

Conclusion

Anthropometric principles and data are intertwined with ergonomics. Therapists need to understand anthropometric concepts so that they may apply anthropometric data to the workplace to optimize job performance, minimize fatigue, and prevent work injuries.

References

Andersson, G.B.J., Ortengren, R. (1974). Lumbar disc pressure and myoelectric back muscle activity during sitting: studies on an office chair. Scandinavian Journal of Rehabilitation Medicine, 3:115-121.

Andersson, G., Ortengren, R., Herberts, P. (1977). Quantitative electromyographic studies of the back muscle activity related to posture and loading. Orthopedic Clinics of North America, 8:85-86.

Armstrong, T.J. (1987). Biomechanical Aspects of Upper Extremity Performance and Disorders. Ann Arbor: University of Michigan Department of Environmental & Industrial Health.

Bjelle, A., Hagber, M., Michaelsson, G. (1979). Clinical and ergonomic factors in prolonged shoulder pain among industrial workers. Scandinavian Journal of Work and Environmental Health, 5:205-206.

Carlett, E.N., and Bishop, R.P. (1976). A technique for assessing postural discomfort. Ergonomics, 19:175.

Chaffin, D. B. (1973). Localized muscle fatigue: Definitions and measurement. Journal of Occupational Medicine, 15:346.

Chaffin, D.B., Anderson, G. (1984). Occupational Biomechanics. New York: Wiley Interscience.

Dullis, R., Contini, R. (1985). Body Segment Parameters (USDEW Office of Vocational Rehabilitation Report No. 1166-03). New York: NYU School of Engineering and Science, 1966. (July 17, 1985; revised April 30, 1986).

Grandjean, E. (1988). Fitting the Task to the Man. London: Taylor & Francis.

Keyserling, W.M. (1986a). A computer aided system to evaluate postural stress in the workplace. American Industrial Hygiene Association Journal, 47:641-644.

Keyserling, W.M. (1986b). Postural analysis of the trunk and shoulders in simulated real time. Ergonomics, 4:569-572.

Keyserling, W.M., Fine, L.J., Punnett, L. (1987). Computer-aided analysis of trunk and shoulder posture. In P. Buckle (Ed.), Musculoskeletal Disorders at Work. London: Taylor & Francis.

Keyserling, W.M., Punnett, L., Fine, L.J. (1988). Trunk posture and back pain: Identification and control of occupational risk factors. Applied Industrial Hygiene, 3:91-92.

Nachemson, A., Morris, J.M. (1964). In vivo measurements of intradiscal pressure. Journal of Bone and Joint Surgery, 46A:1077-1078.

National Aeronautics and Space Administration (1978). Anthropometric Source Book. Volume 1: Anthropometry for Designers. (Publ. No. 1024). Washington, D.C.: NASA.

National Institute for Occupational Health and Safety (1981). Work Practices Guide for Manual Lifting. DHHS (NIOSH) Publ. No. 81-122. Cincinnati: United States Government Printing Office.

Van Wely, P. (1970). Design and disease. Applied Ergonomics, 1:262.

CHAPTER 3

Basic Biomechanics

Laurie A. Vincello

ABSTRACT

The purpose of this chapter is to help the reader to gain a basic understanding of the principles of biomechanics. The biomechanical model uses the laws of physics to explain motion of the body segments and the forces that act on these body segments. This chapter explains how to use functional units in analysis. It then uses the model to solve basic problems that involve the upper extremity, the trunk, and hand grip. Readers can use this information to increase their knowledge of person-machine systems and to aid in the design of rehabilitation programs.

An understanding of biomechanics is necessary to understand the laws that govern movement of the human body. The biomechanical model allows one to estimate the forces that act on different component structures and sometimes to predict the maximum allowable magnitude for a load held in various postures, the appropriate size of tools, and the least stressful configuration of the workplace (Chaffin & Anderson, 1984). The practical application of these principles maximizes performance, conserves energy, and prevents skeletal disorders in industry. In the workplace, person and machine systems are designed with biomechanics in mind (Grandjean, 1988). "Biomechanics uses laws of physics and engineering concepts to describe motion undergone by the various body part segments and the forces acting on these body parts during normal daily activities" (Frankel & Nordin, 1980, p. ix). This chapter is only a brief overview of the field of biomechanics. Many texts on this subject offer methods for multidimensional and dynamic analysis that are not discussed here.

There are two areas of study in biomechanics: statics and dynamics. Statics is the study of a body at rest or equilibrium. Dynamics is the study of moving bodies. Dynamics involves kinematics, which examines the relationship between displacement, velocity, and acceleration in transitional or rotational motion, and kinetics, which involves moving bodies and the forces on them that produce motion (LeVeau, 1992).

Anatomy

It is important to understand the composition and function of the tissues involved in body mechanics. The following is a review of tissues and structures.

Bone

In biomechanics the important mechanical properties of bone are strength and stiffness. Loading the bone causes temporary deformation unless the load is excessive and goes beyond the elastic stage into the plastic phase, which leads to failure. Bone is subjected to many types of loading, including tension, compression, bending, shear, torsion, and any combination of these forces.

Tension occurs when equal and opposite forces are applied inward from the surface of the structure. The structure lengthens and narrows as tension is applied. Compression force exists when equal and opposite loads are applied toward the surface of the structure. In this case the structure shortens and widens. Shear force is applied parallel to the structure and deforms the structure in an angular manner. Bending is a combination of tension and compression. The loads are applied to cause the structure to bend around an axis. Therefore, tension occurs on the convex side and compression on the concave side of the structure. Torsion occurs when the forces applied cause the structure to twist around an axis. Living bone seldom experiences a load in one mode, so it is therefore subjected to a combination of these loads (Nordin & Frankel, 1989). When a structure has been injured and is healing, the maximum loads that the structure can withstand may be altered. So, the therapist may need to modify a task or progressively increase the intensity of a task to match the ability of the structure to withstand the load.

Tendons and Ligaments

Tendons transmit tensile loads from muscle to bone, causing joint movement. Ligaments provide stability; they guide motion and prevent excessive motion. According to physiologic studies (Nordin & Frankel, 1989, p.65), in normal conditions, these structures are subjected to a stress magnitude only one-third of the maximum stress they can withstand. In normal circumstances these structures undergo deformation and recovery. "Residual strain" occurs when a tendon or ligament is subjected to repeated stretch with insufficient recovery time (Chaffin, 1984). The tendon or ligament may elongate 1 to 2% of its no-load length. This leads to weakening, inflammation, and decreased function. There is a need for additional research in this area. If the maximum stress value of a structure is exceeded, complete, rapid failure occurs with loss of load-bearing ability.

Skeletal Muscle

Muscles provide strength and protection to the skeleton by distributing loads and absorbing shock. They perform both static work, to maintain posture, and dynamic work, for locomotion and positioning in space. The maximum amount of contractile tension is achieved when the muscle is halfway between its shortest and longest lengths. This position is called the resting length. The ability of the muscle to produce contractile tension decreases as the muscle shortens or lengthens beyond the resting length. In a concentric contraction, the greater the external load, the slower is the velocity of movement. When the external load reaches the maximum force that a muscle can exert, the velocity becomes zero; this is called an isometric contraction, and the muscle is in biomechanical equilibrium. When the external load exceeds the maximum muscular force, the contraction is eccentric. In an eccentric contraction, the greater the external load, the faster is the velocity of movement. In the force-velocity relationship, the slower the muscle contracts, the greater is the internal muscular tension, and the faster the muscle contracts, the less is the internal muscular tension (Nordin & Frankel, 1989) (Table 3–1).

Principles of Physics

Vectors

Linear vectors lie in the same line of application as each other. These vectors simply add together to equal the resultant vector (Figure 3–1).

Concurrent vectors are two vectors that act on the same body part in different directions. Two-dimensional models are used to examine them. Concurrent vectors can be resolved into a single vector called the resultant vector by means of the parallelogram method or by mathematics (Figure 3–2).

The parallelogram method involves drawing the concurrent vectors, represented by 3N and 4N in Figure 3–2, that originate from the same point. Lines are then drawn parallel to the concurrent vectors starting at the end points of the vectors, illustrated by the dashed lines in Figure 3–2. The resultant vector, C, is drawn from the original starting point and ends at the intersection of the two lines that were drawn parallel to the concurrent vectors. The value of C in newtons is its length in the drawing.

TABLE 3–1   Mathematical Relationships

Space:	length is measured in meters, area in square meters, and volume in liters.
Time:	is measured in seconds.
Matter:	is that which occupies space.
Mass:	is the quantity of an object. It is measured in kilograms.
Vector:	is a line that has quantity and direction. It indicates displacement.
Displacement:	indicates the difference between the initial position and the ending position.
Acceleration:	is the final velocity minus the initial velocity divided by time: $$\frac{V_f - V_i}{t}$$
Weight:	is measured in newtons. It is equal to mass multiplied by gravity: $W = ma$.
Force:	is that which causes movement. It is measured in newtons. Forces can be compressive—directed toward the surface; tensile—directed away from the surface; shear or tangential—directed parallel to the surface.
Stress:	is found within the material the forces are acting upon. It is measured in newtons per meter squared: $\frac{N}{m^2}$ It is determined by multiplying the force times the specific quantity of that tissue.
Friction:	is determined by the normal force multiplied by the coefficient of friction for that particular material.
Lifting Work:	is defined as weight (mass × gravity) multiplied by height multiplied by number of repetitions: $Lw = (m)\ (a)\ (h)\ (r)$.
Gravity:	is a constant and is defined as the rate of acceleration in proportion to the square root of the distance traveled. The earth's gravity equals 9.8 m/sec^2; for the purposes of this chapter, it is rounded to 10 m/sec^2 (Roberts & Falkenburg, 1992).

The Pythagorean theorem is used to calculate the length of the resultant vector C with mathematics. The theorem states that in a right triangle the sum of the sides squared equals the hypotenuse squared:

$$a^2 + b^2 = c^2$$

In Figure 3-2

$$3^2 + 4^2 = C^2$$

$$9 + 16 = C^2$$

$$25 = C^2$$

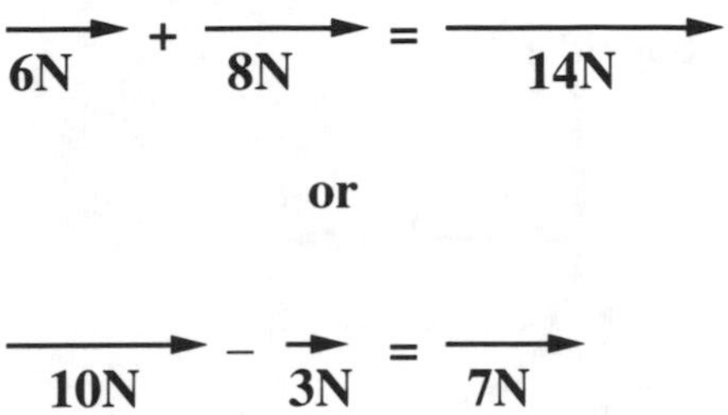

$$\overrightarrow{6N} + \overrightarrow{8N} = \overrightarrow{14N}$$

or

$$\overrightarrow{10N} - \overrightarrow{3N} = \overrightarrow{7N}$$

Figure 3–1 Linear vectors. The therapist uses simple mathematics to obtain the value of the resultant vector.

$$\sqrt{25} = C$$
$$5 = C$$

so the value of vector C is 5 N (or *newtons*).

Circular Relationships

Circular relationships exist when movement takes place around a fixed axis such as a joint. The force that travels around the axis is called the moment. The distance from the axis to a location perpendicular to the point of application of the force is called the moment arm. An example of a circular relationship is that between the elbow joint and a force at the middle of the forearm (Figure 3–3).

The length of the moment arm at the range of motion depicted in Figure 3–3 is represented by d. The length of the moment arm changes instant to instant throughout the range of motion. The length of d is longest when the elbow is at 90 degrees of flexion and shortest when the elbow is in full extension.

In Figure 3–3, L represents the lever arm, which is the distance along a body part from the axis to the point of application of the force. L remains constant throughout the range of motion. The lever is the rigid body that

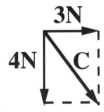

Figure 3–2 Concurrent vectors. Use of the parallelogram method or the Pythagorean theorem to obtain the value of the resultant vector C.

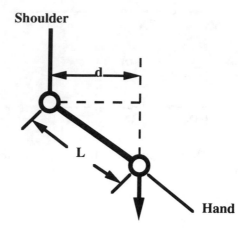

Figure 3–3   Circular relationship. The moment arm is represented by d and the lever arm by L.

moves around an axis. In the example the lever arm is the bones of the forearm.

Equilibrium is the condition in which the forces in one direction equal the forces in the opposite direction. Figure 3–4 depicts a seesaw arrangement. The goal is to keep the seesaw level, in equilibrium; that is, the sum of the forces equals zero ($\Sigma F = 0$).

In this problem the force X required to keep the seesaw from moving must be calculated. The forces to the left of the fulcrum equal the force (5N) multiplied by the lever arm (10m).

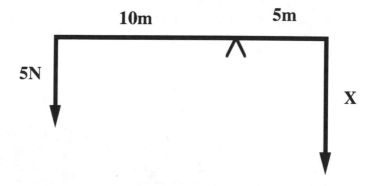

Figure 3–4   A state of equilibrium. The forces on each side of the fulcrum are equal.

Therefore,

$$F = (5N) \times (10m)$$

The forces to the right of the fulcrum equal the force (X) multiplied by the length of the lever arm (5m), so

$$F = (X) \times (5m)$$

To calculate $\Sigma F = 0$

$$(5N)(10m) - (XN)(5m) = 0$$

$$(5N)(10m) = (XN)(5m)$$

$$50Nm = 5XNm$$

$$50 \frac{Nm}{5m} = XN$$

$$10 = X$$

So, the force required by X to keep this seesaw from tipping equals 10 N.

Figure 3–4 depicts an example of a first-class lever, in which the axis lies between the two forces. An example in the human body is the triceps brachii muscle. A second-class lever is that in which the resistance is between the effort force and the axis. An example of such a lever is a wheelbarrow or the gastrocnemius and soleus muscles when a person raises him- or herself up onto his or her toes while standing. A third-class lever is that in which the effort force is located between the axis and the resistance. An example of this type of lever is the biceps brachii muscle and most of the musculoskeletal levers. The best mechanical advantage exists when the effort arm, the distance from the axis to the effort, is longer than the resistance arm, the distance from the axis to the resistance. This condition exists in a second-class lever. It is also the reason for a person to keep a load close, to reduce the length of the resistance arm. Because most levers in the human body are third-class levers, the body is not efficient and requires muscular effort several times greater than the weight of the object lifted. Tools and proper positioning can minimize this effect (Yates & Lindberg, 1970).

In addition to levers two other musculoskeletal arrangements provide movement. The first is similar to a wheel-and-axle arrangement. An example in the human body is medial rotation of the humerus around the longitudinal axis of the humerus. The other type is a pulley arrangement. An example is the pulling of the patella between the condyles of the femur during knee extension (White & Panjabi, 1990).

Center of Gravity

The center of gravity of an object is defined as the point within the body where the total mass of the body is concentrated. If a body rests on its center of gravity, it is in equilibrium (White & Panjabi, 1990). The center of gravity of a human body resting in an erect posture is just anterior to the first sacral vertebra. That location is approximately at the level of 55% of the height of a person. Therapists are taught that increasing the base of support increases the stability of clients. The goal is to lower the center of gravity and to keep it positioned over the base of support. When the center of gravity falls outside the base of support, equilibrium is lost. The center of gravity does not always remain within the body. In a quadruped stance, the center of gravity falls outside the body just anterior to the pelvic region, but because the center of gravity is within the base of support, this is a stable stance (Rasch & Burke, 1978). Each body segment has a center of gravity, and its location is used when calculating the forces acting upon that body segment.

Torque

Torque is the amount of force required to produce a rotation around an axis. It is expressed as mass multiplied by acceleration multiplied by the moment arm ($F = ma \times$ moment arm). The units for torque are newton-meters or foot-pounds. External torque is the weight of the body segment multiplied by the moment arm. Internal torque is that produced around a joint by muscles, tendons, and other soft tissues. Internal torque is equal to the force of the muscular contraction multiplied by the moment arm. The values of both external and internal torque change throughout the range of motion because of the change in the length of the moment arm.

Biomechanical Relationships

Trunk

Back pain has three causes—abnormal strain on a normal back; normal stress on an abnormal back; and normal stress on a normal back unprepared for the stress. Abnormal strain on a normal back becomes painful during a prolonged lift. Muscle fatigue puts stress on the ligaments, which eventually fail, forcing the joints to take the load. Pain arises from muscular ischemia, excessive strain on the ligaments, or capsular stretch. Normal strain on an abnormal back occurs when a structural abnormality exists, such as scoliosis, tight hamstrings, or tight lumbar spinal muscles. These conditions cause a shift in the center of gravity and therefore a reduction in the efficiency of the lift. Normal stress on an unprepared back occurs with improper anticipation of the weight of a load to be lifted or with a fatigued back, both of which cause improper positioning (Caillet, 1988).

The biomechanical functional unit of the trunk is the vertebral column. It provides the framework on which the body and the extremities move. From cervical to lumbar regions the structures become larger, and the direction of the articular surfaces changes. The parts of the vertebrae are as follows. The body is the main load-bearing section; the pedicles form the neural arch; the four facets on each vertebra have different orientations and direct the movement at that level; the spinous and transverse processes provide muscle attachments (White & Panjabi, 1990). Eighty-five to ninety-five percent of all disk herniations occur at L4-5 and L5-S1 in equal frequency. The L5-S1 disk is chosen to represent lumbar stress during lifting because it incurs the largest moment during lifting because of the long moment arm relative to a load in the hands (Chaffin & Anderson, 1984).

Figure 3–5 shows the solution to a basic lifting problem. A person is holding a box that weighs 15 kg. The center of gravity of the box is 0.2 m ventral to the center of motion of the L5-S1 disk. The force of the weight of the upper body passes 0.02 m dorsal to the transverse axis of motion of the L5-S1 disk. The weight of the upper body is 40 kg. One must determine how much force (F) the erector spinae muscles must exert if the moment arm is 0.04 m.

The therapist first calculates the forces exerted by the box and upper body by multiplying mass by acceleration (F = ma). Acceleration in this example is equal to the force of gravity (10 m/s^2) because the person is stationary. The force exerted by the box equals 15 kg × 10 m/s^2 = 150 N. The force exerted by the upper body equals 40 kg × 10 m/s^2 = 400 N. The sum of the forces must equal zero to maintain the lift. The sum of the forces is found by multiplying the force by the length of the moment arm

$$(150N \times 0.2m) - (400N \times 0.02m) - (F \times 0.04m) = 0$$

$$(150N \times 0.2m) - (400N \times 0.02m) = F \times 0.04m$$

$$\frac{(30Nm - 8Nm)}{0.04m} = F$$

$$550N = F$$

Therefore, the erector spinae muscles must exert a force of 550 N to maintain this lift. If the box were held farther from the body, the moment arm for the box would be larger, and the force exerted by the erector spinae muscles would be greater. This is why clients are taught to keep the load close during a lift or carry. The goal is to keep the moment arm as short as possible and therefore the muscular effort as small as possible. To calculate the reaction force on the L5-S1 disk, one again uses the formula ΣF = 0. The forces of gravity of the box, upper body, and erector spinae muscles all pull downward; the reaction force on the L5-S1 disk must be upward of equal magnitude. The reaction force on the disk is represented by D as follows:

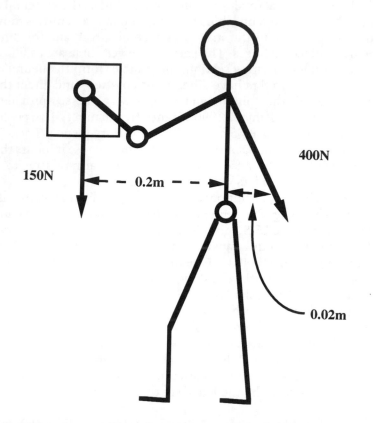

Figure 3–5   Lifting. Box weighs 15 kg. Its center of gravity is 0.2 m ventral to L5-S1 disk. Upper body weighs 40 kg and passes 0.02 m dorsal to L5-S1 disk.

$$0 = D - 150N - 400N - 550N$$

$$D = 50N + 400N + 550N$$

$$D = 1100N$$

So, the reaction force on the L5-S1 disk equals 1100 N.

Controversy exists over the proper lifting form. Research by Wiktorin and Nordin (1986) demonstrated that compressive forces on the disk do not lead to rupture, and the authors advocated the squat and lift technique. Other research indicates that when an object is too large to straddle, stooping over the object to lift it produces less compressive force than the squat and lift technique. However, the shear forces are greater in the stooped posture, so maintaining an erect torso is preferred. Unfortunately, the best lordotic posture has not yet been determined and requires more research (Chaffin & Anderson, 1984).

Upper Extremity

There are five functional units in the upper extremity: the shoulder girdle, the shoulder joint, the elbow, the radioulnar joint, and the wrist and hand. These units are designed for either stability or mobility.

Shoulder girdle

The shoulder girdle complex is designed for mobility. It consists of the clavicle and the scapula and their articulations. The sternoclavicular joint has little stability. It is the site of the most movement and acts as an axis for rotation of the shoulder girdle. It also absorbs lateral shock. The acromio-clavicular joint is weak and absorbs the stress of impacts on the shoulder. The muscles of the shoulder girdle provide stability because the bony and ligamentous arrangements are weak. A lack of upper body strength is a factor in a great number of injuries (White & Panjabi, 1990).

Shoulder joint

The shoulder joint consists of the glenoid fossa and the head of the humerus. It is a multiaxial joint that is designed for mobility because at any given time less than one-half of the head of the humerus is in the socket. The rotator cuff muscles and the labrum offer stability.

The following is a description of the function of the muscles that cross the shoulder joint. The infraspinatus and teres minor muscles insert on the posterior aspect of the humerus. They are arranged in a wheel-and-axle mechanism to cause lateral rotation of the humerus around a longitudinal axis. The subscapularis muscle inserts on the anterior aspect of the head of the humerus. It also functions in a wheel-and-axle manner, causing medial rotation of the humerus around a longitudinal axis. The supraspinatus muscle inserts on the distal aspect of the head of the humerus above the anterior posterior axis of rotation of the shoulder joint. It is a first-class lever mechanism that pulls the head of the humerus medially to allow for abduction of the humerus. The latissimus dorsi and teres major muscles originate on the posterior trunk and insert on the anterior aspect of the humerus. They are arranged in a wheel-and-axle formation to cause medial rotation and extension of the humerus (White & Panjabi, 1990).

Elbow joint

The elbow joint consists of the distal end of the humerus, the proximal end of the ulna, and the proximal end of the radius. The humeral-ulnar arrangement is designed for stability, but the humeral-radial joint is weak. Continual

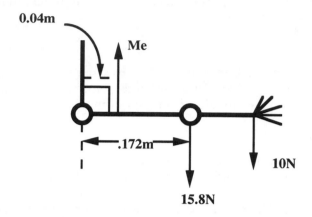

Figure 3–6   Elbow at 90 degrees, 1-kg weight at the wrist.

excessive stress at the humeral-radioulnar area is common and leads to injury.

The main elbow flexors are the biceps, brachialis, and brachioradialis muscles. Elbow extension is achieved by the action of the triceps brachii muscle. The other muscles act as stabilizers because their lines of force pass so closely to the elbow joint that they generate only small rotary torques (White & Panjabi, 1990).

Radioulnar joint

The radioulnar joint consists of proximal, distal, and middle joints. It lacks bony stability, so the ligaments provide stability. The movements are supination and pronation around a longitudinal axis. The biceps brachii muscle has a wheel-and-axle arrangement that causes supination. The supinator muscle provides stability and assists in supination. The pronator teres and pronator quadratus muscles provide stability in adduction to cause pronation (White & Panjabi, 1990).

The muscular effort required by the biceps muscle to maintain different angles of the elbow joint is calculated in the following example. A person has a 1-kg weight around the wrist. The length of the forearm is 0.3 m. The center of gravity of the forearm is 0.172 m below the elbow joint. The arm weighs 1.58 kg. First, one calculates the value of the muscular effort required with the forearm at a 90-degree angle relative to the upper arm. The values used for center of gravity and arm weight are for the average man based on anthropometric measurements (Figure 3–6).

The force exerted by the forearm itself is calculated with the formula F = ma. So, F = (1.58 kg) × (10 m/s). Therefore, F = 15.8 N. The force exerted by the weight at the wrist is F = (1 kg) × (10 m/s) = 10 N. To calculate the muscular

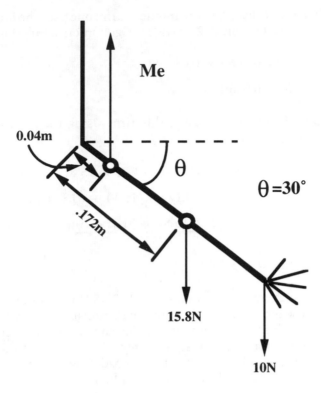

Figure 3–7 Elbow at angle 30 degrees below horizontal. The moment arm is the distance from the axis to a line perpendicular to the line of force.

effort (Me) required by the biceps to keep the forearm at a 90-degree angle, one begins with the formula $\Sigma F = 0$

$$0 = (\text{Me} \times 0.04\text{m}) - (0.172\text{m} \times 15.8\text{N}) - (0.3\text{m} \times 10\text{N})$$

$$(\text{Me} \times 0.04\text{m}) = (0.172 \times 15.8) + (0.3 \times 10)$$

$$\text{Me} = \frac{[(0.172 \times 15.8) + (0.3 \times 10)]}{0.04}$$

$$\text{Me} = 142.9\text{N}$$

So the biceps exerts a force of 142.9 N in an upward direction to maintain this position.

The muscular effort required with the forearm 30 degrees below horizontal is calculated in Figure 3–7. All other values remain unchanged.

To calculate the length of the moment arm, one uses the formula cosine 30 degrees = X / 0.04 (Table 3–2 provides trigonometric functions).

$$X = 0.8660 \times 0.04$$

$$X = 0.035m$$

The sum of the forces is zero, this time using the new value for the length of the moment arm

$$O = (Me \times 0.035) - (0.172 \times 15.8) - (0.3 \times 10)$$

$$Me \times 0.035 = (0.172 \times 15.8) + (0.3 \times 10)$$

$$Me = \frac{[(0.172 \times 15.8) + (0.3 \times 10)]}{0.035}$$

$$Me = 163.36N$$

The biceps must exert an upward force of 163.36 N to maintain the forearm 30 degrees below horizontal. This example demonstrates how the muscular effort changes with the range of motion. The shorter the moment arm, as in Figure 3–7, the greater is the muscular effort required to lift the same load. This is why it is possible to carry a heavy load at waist level but to find it difficult, or impossible, to place it on a shelf higher than waist height.

Wrist joint

The wrist joint consists of the distal ends of the radius and ulna and the carpal bones. The movements are flexion, extension, radial deviation, and ulnar deviation. The bony arrangements lack stability, so stability is provided by the ligaments and the tendons (White & Panjabi, 1990).

The hand

Problems can arise in the workplace if the wrong type of grip is used. There is a great difference in the forces required by the flexor digitorum profundus muscles in partial-hand-grip and in whole-hand grip. The forces required by the flexor digitorum profundus muscle to maintain the grip are calculated in the following example. The object grasped is 0.085 m in diameter, and maintaining the grip requires 3 kg of pressure. In both types of grasp, the thumb is abducted to 70 degrees. In the partial-hand grip the force is applied at an 80-degree angle to the tendon and contact is made at the distal phalanges. In the whole-hand grip the force is applied at a 50-degree angle. The tendons are 0.005 m from the axis of motion of the finger joints.

TABLE 3–2: Trigonometric Functions*

Degrees	Sines	Cosines	Tangents	Cotangents	
0	.0000	1.0000	.0000		90
1	.0175	.9998	.0175	57.290	89
2	.0349	.9994	.0349	28.636	88
3	.0523	.9986	.0524	19.081	87
4	.0698	.9976	.0699	14.301	86
5	.0872	.9962	.0875	11.430	85
6	.1045	.9945	.1051	9.5144	84
7	.1219	.9925	.1228	8.1443	83
8	.1392	.9903	.1405	7.1154	82
9	.1564	.9877	.1584	6.3138	81
10	.1736	.9848	.1763	5.6713	80
11	.1908	.9816	.1944	5.1446	79
12	.2079	.9781	.2126	4.7046	78
13	.2250	.9744	.2309	4.3315	77
14	.2419	.9703	.2493	4.0108	76
15	.2588	.9659	.2679	3.7321	75
16	.2756	.9613	.2867	3.4874	74
17	.2924	.9563	.3057	3.2709	73
18	.3090	.9511	.3249	3.0777	72
19	.3256	.9455	.3443	2.9042	71
20	.3420	.9397	.3640	2.7475	70
21	.3584	.9336	.3839	2.6051	69
22	.3746	.9272	.4040	2.4751	68
23	.3907	.9205	.4245	2.3559	67
24	.4067	.9135	.4452	2.2460	66
25	.4226	.9063	.4663	2.1445	65
26	.4384	.8988	.4877	2.0503	64
27	.4540	.8910	.5095	1.9626	63
28	.4695	.8829	.5317	1.8807	62
29	.4848	.8746	.5543	1.8040	61
30	.5000	.8660	.5774	1.7321	60
31	.5150	.8572	.6009	1.6643	59
32	.5299	.8480	.6249	1.6003	58
33	.5446	.8387	.6494	1.5399	57
34	.5592	.8290	.6745	1.4826	56
35	.5736	.8192	.7002	1.4281	55
36	.5878	.8090	.7265	1.3765	54
37	.6018	.7986	.7536	1.3270	53
38	.6157	.7880	.7813	1.2799	52
39	.6293	.7771	.8098	1.2349	51
40	.6428	.7660	.8391	1.1918	50
41	.6561	.7547	.8693	1.1504	49
42	.6691	.7431	.9004	1.1106	48
43	.6820	.7314	.9325	1.0724	47
44	.6947	.7193	.9657	1.0355	46
45	.7071	.7071	1.0000	1.0000	45
	Cosines	Sines	Cotangents	Tangents	Degrees

*Note: With angles above 45 degrees be sure to see the headings that appear at the bottom of the columns. (Roberts & Falkenburg, 1992)

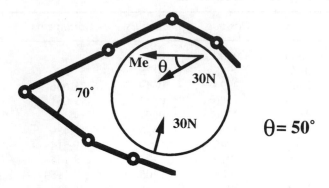

Figure 3–8 Whole-hand grip. Most of hand in contact with object.

The formula used to calculate the muscular effort required is as follows (see also Figure 3–8; Appendix 3–1):

$$\cos 50 \text{ degrees} = \frac{30N}{Me}$$

$$Me = \frac{30N}{\cos 50 \text{ degrees}}$$

$$Me = \frac{30}{0.6428}$$

$$Me = 46.7N$$

In the whole-hand grip, a force of 46.7 N is required to grasp this object.

The same formula is used to calculate the muscular effort in partial-hand grip (Figure 3–9; Appendix 3–1).

$$\cos 80 \text{ degrees} = \frac{30N}{Me}$$

$$Me = \frac{30}{\cos 80 \text{ degrees}}$$

$$Me = \frac{30}{0.1736}$$

$$Me = 172.8N$$

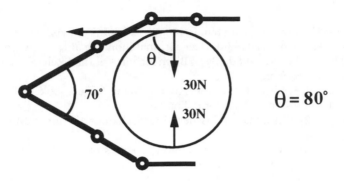

Figure 3–9   Partial-hand grip. Contact at thumb and distal phalanges.

So to use a partial-hand grip requires a force of 172.8 N instead of the 46.7 N required by a whole-hand grip. Therefore, using the partial-hand grip requires nearly four times the force of using a whole-hand grip. This is important in the evaluation of factors that contribute to carpal tunnel problems (Roberts & Falkenburg, 1992).

Conclusion

Biomechanics explains the actions achieved by the human body. Knowledge of biomechanics led to design criteria for seating for aircraft pilots and office workers; the establishment of permissible control forces and locations in aircraft and the cabs of industrial cranes and of turning lathes and other machines; limits for loads to be lifted and carried in various postures; and design guides for hand tools (Shackel, 1976). Limits exist for actions that can be performed by the human body, and guidelines reflect these limits. The guidelines can be obtained from the National Institute for Occupational Safety and Health (NIOSH).

This chapter is a brief discussion of biomechanics in light of the breadth of information available and the research being conducted. The examples in this chapter are for illustrative purposes only and do not necessarily reflect real-life situations. The information is meant to expose therapists to the field of biomechanics to enhance their knowledge of person-machine interactions and to aid them in designing rehabilitation programs. To make computations for a specific client, the therapist should consult a book that focuses on problem-solving methods.

References

Caillet, R. (1988). Low Back Pain Syndrome. Philadelphia: Davis.

Chaffin, D.B., Anderson, G. (1984). Occupational Biomechanics. New York: Wiley.

Frankel, V.H., Nordin, M. (1980). Basic Biomechanics of the Skeletal System. Philadelphia: Lea & Febiger.

Grandjean, E. (1988). Fitting the Task to the Man: A Textbook of Occupational Biomechanics. London: Taylor & Francis.

LeVeau, B.F. (1992). Williams and Lissner's Biomechanics of Human Motion, 3rd ed. Philadelphia: Saunders.

Nordin, M., Frankel, V.H. (1989). Basic Biomechanics of the Musculoskeletal Systems. Philadelphia: Lea & Febiger.

Rasch, P.J., Burke, R.K. (1978). Kinesiology and Applied Anatomy. Philadelphia: Lea & Febiger.

Roberts, S.L., Falkenburg, S.A. (1992). Biomechanics: Problem Solving for Functional Activity. St. Louis: Mosby Year Book.

Shackel, B. (1976). Applied Ergonomics Handbook. Vol. 3. Guilford, England: IPC.

White, A.A. III, Panjabi, M.M. (1990). Clinical Biomechanics of the Spine. Philadelphia: Lippincott.

Wiktorin, C.H., Nordin, M. (1986). Introduction to Problem Solving in Biomechanics. Philadelphia: Lea & Febiger.

Yates, J.A., Lundberg, A.C. (1970). Moving and Lifting Patients: Principles and Techniques. Minneapolis: Sister Kenny Institute.

Suggested Reading

Fritjof, C. (1984). The Tao of Physics. New York: Bantam.

Fung, Y.C. (1990). Biomechanics—Motion, Flow, Stress and Growth. New York: Springer-Verlag.

Fung, Y.C.B. (1967). Stress-strain-history relations of soft tissues in simple elongation. American Journal of Physiology, 213:1532-1544.

Hall, S.J. (1991). Basic Biomechanics. St. Louis: Mosby Year Book.

Holder, L.I. (1984). College Algebra and Trigonometry, 3rd ed. Belmont, Calif: Wadsworth.

Special thanks to my husband, David, for his support and understanding; to my children, Stephanie and Timothy, for their love and patience; and to Kathleen Ryan, PT, for her assistance.

Appendix 3–1

Trigonometric Functions

For a right triangle

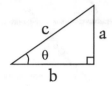

$$\text{Sin} = \frac{a}{c} \qquad\qquad \text{CSC} = \frac{C}{a}$$

$$\text{COS} = \frac{b}{c} \qquad\qquad \text{SEC} = \frac{C}{b}$$

$$\tan = \frac{a}{b} \qquad\qquad \cot = \frac{b}{a}$$

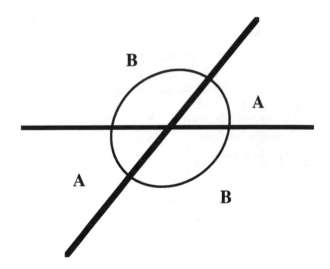

Supplementary angles: A line intersected by another line forms two angles, which when added together equal 180 degrees. Therefore, A + B = 180 degrees.

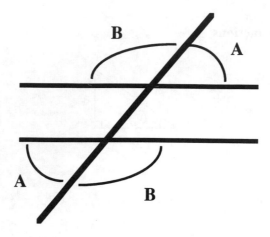

Alternate angles: When two parallel lines are intersected by a third line, the angles on opposite sides of the intersecting lines will be equal. Therefore, angles A are equal, and angles B are equal.

Pythagorean Theorem

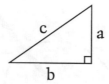

$$a^2 + b^2 = C^2$$

In a right triangle the sum of the sides squared equals the hypotenuse squared. (Source: Holder, L.I. [1984]. College Algebra and Trigonometry, 3rd ed. Belmont, Calif.: Wadsworth.)

CHAPTER 4

Cognitive Workload

David J. Folts, A. James Giannini, and Bonnie Otonicar

ABSTRACT

Cognitive workload is defined as a worker's perception of the work being completed in relation to the workplace. This chapter focuses on areas that affect cognitive workload and provides evaluation tools that can be used in industry for measuring cognitive workload.

The term *ergonomics* is of Greek origin and means "work law." Although he did not use the term, Frederick Taylor (Sanders & McCormick, 1987) performed detailed studies that provided the foundation for ergonomic study. Taylor emphasized that one must observe, measure, and study human behavior during work if there is to be an improvement in organizational efficiency. These studies showed a large variation in the performance capacity of workers. A therapist who works in ergonomics strives to develop the best match between a worker and the attributes of his or her job. The therapist is concerned with the physical and mental interactions required to perform a task.

The evaluation of cognitive workload is one approach to the study of ergonomics. *Cognitive workload* is defined as a worker's perception of the work being performed or the difficulty perceived in the work. Cognitive workload also encompasses information-processing by the worker. Cognitive workload is a useful tool for therapists because the important measurement is frequently not the work being completed but the work being perceived.

The intensity at which a person chooses to work depends on cognitive workload (Gamberale, 1988).

To understand a worker, a therapist studies not only the worker's physical performance but also the worker's perception of the workload. A worker's perception of the workload may differ from the employer's perception, and this lack of agreement may lead to work-related injuries (Gallagher, 1991; Kuronski, 1991). It has been noted that an individual's perception of work tolerance frequently does not correspond with the capacity of work measured (Fiori, 1991; Luczah, 1991; Tsang & Johnson, 1989).

First Studies of Cognitive Workload

The initial studies dealt with general psychophysical problems of subjective force and cognitive workload. The early results showed that the perception of applied force followed a positively accelerating function. In other words, in many different dimensions of physical work, the subjective intensity grows according to the physical load (Hermansen & Saltin, 1956; Stevens, 1962).

The rating of cognitive workload historically has been accomplished by means of biopsychophysical categories. Extroversion-introversion has been evaluated with the Minnesota Multiphasic Personality Inventory (MMPI) and the Eysenck Personality Inventory (Eysenck, 1962), somatic perception with the Somatic Perception Questionnaire (Frankenhaeser et al, 1969), anxiety with the Speilberger state-trait inventory (Gillet & Morgan, 1977), and depression with the Beck Depression Inventory (Luce, 1972). One of the most useful methods of estimating the magnitude of cognitive workload in muscular work was developed by Borg (1982). The scale is based on one's rating perceived exertion from extremely light to extremely heavy. The task of the person performing the work is to assign a value to the subjective sensation of work being performed.

Principles of Cognitive Workload

A knowledge of workload measurement is essential to therapists who use ergonomics in their practices. However, many studies that have attempted to compare workload measurements have been inconsistent and disappointing. Two techniques that have proved useful include the Subjective Workload Assessment Technique (SWAT) and the National Aeronautics and Space Administration (NASA) Test Load Index (TLX) test.

The SWAT (Reid & Nygren, 1988) was devised to provide a measurement of mental workload that is based on three criteria. The measurements include psychologic stress and load, mental load, and time load. The SWAT uses a conjoint measurement method. To evaluate the validity of workload judgment, the SWAT requires a factual presentation of the three areas of measurement (3 × 3 × 3 design). These combinations do not have to be a complete set for proper workload measurement. In the scale development phase of the SWAT, the workload combinations are rank ordered. Next, a series of statistical tests are used to determine factors such as the relations between time, effort, and stress and whether or not the rank ordering is proper. Contradictions when found are usually specific to one dimension, reflecting that the rater treats the dimension as meaningless or that the dimension has no effect on workload. The modified rank data are then rescaled to determine the best-fitting scale.

The second phase of SWAT is called event scoring. Dimensions are represented by all three point scales. After a task has been evaluated, the rater provides a verbal judgment for the three dimensions that reflects the perceived loading that has been experienced in each dimension. The event scores are then transmitted to individual component scores of time, effort, and stress, which are then added to provide an overall workload score.

The NASA TLX (Hart & Staveland, 1988) is a multifactorial rating scale that has been shown to be sensitive to changes in operator levels of workload in many different contexts. Workload score is based on weighted averages of the following dimensions: mental demands, physical demands, temporal demands, performance, effort, and frustration. Similar to the SWAT, the evaluation is based on a two-part procedure. After workers have completed a group of tasks, importance estimates of the six dimensions are obtained. The six factors are presented to the worker with 15 paired comparisons. The worker circles the member of each pair that he or she believes contributes more than the other to the workload of the task. The number of times each dimension is chosen in a pair is then counted (valued from 0 to 5), and this number is placed in a range from 0.00 to 0.33 so that the sum of the weight is 1.0. These weights are then used to produce a relative rank ordering of the associated importance of each task. A continuous 12-cm time scale is presented on a video display or by paper and pencil to display numerical ratings on six 20-point rating scales. Each scale is then multiplied by a factor of 5 so that each of the six new scales ranges from 0 to 100. The rated values of each of the six dimensions are then added to show an overall workload estimate.

Cognitive Overload

Various demands that workers encounter while working relate to different kinds of stimulus overloads (Gopher & Dauchin, 1986). Overload can be defined as the worker's lack of capacity to tolerate incoming perceptual signals. In other words, a lack of sensory integration occurs because of overload. Overload occurs when the total amount of work exceeds what the worker can accomplish during a specified period. Researchers have determined that perceived job exertion correlates with quantitative and qualitative overload (Frankenhaeser & Gardell, 1976). French and Calplan found that overloaded workers displayed lower self concept, larger numbers of task errors, higher heart rates, and higher cholesterol levels than workers who were not overloaded. Perceptions of high job demands have a negative effect on satisfaction and greatly increase psychologic stress (French & Calplan, 1972).

Type A and Type B Personality Moderators

The degree of pressure on a worker to perform also acts as a moderator (Karase, 1979). This measurement is analogous to the Type A behavioral pattern described by Friedman and Rosenman (Thurstone, 1951). A Type A worker displays a behavioral pattern that demonstrates a sense of urgency and striving. Friedman found that this activity level demonstrates the highest correlation with Type A behavioral patterns (Friedman & Rosenman, 1974). Workers with a high activity level have a weak negative relationship between perceived job demands and satisfaction. Type A workers have been shown to overload themselves on purpose by taking on an everincreasing number of activities (Rosenman, 1980). Thus, workers with a high activity level are less likely than those with a low activity level to report cognitive overload in highly demanding work situations. Additional research (Giannini et al, 1978; Miller et al, 1977; Wickens, 1984) has shown that the relationship between workload and stress is greater for workers with Type A personalities than for those with Type B behavioral characteristics. A high cognitive workload may cause a worker to perceive that he or she will not meet expectations, which causes even greater stress than the cognitive overload itself.

Cognitive Workload: Practical Applications

Job tasks place demands on workers' cognitive workloads. Even when there is task repetition in a job, the worker is constantly processing information and making decisions based on this feedback system (Armstrong et al, 1984; Ulin et al, 1990; Ulin et al, in press). Cognitive workload can be divided into the following areas.

Perception

Perception is the manner in which workers collect information using their five senses. In the industrial setting, information is transmitted through displays such as gauges, dials, video monitors, alarms, and sirens. In a broad sense, a display can be considered any source of information that is received through the five senses.

Tables 4–1 through 4–7 may be used by therapists to conduct a job analysis in an industrial setting. The reason for the analysis may be to gain information about the job of a client who is undergoing work hardening or to provide a company with information on how it can improve workstations in terms of safety and productivity. The "Standards of Practice for Occupational Therapy" (Shriver & Foto, 1983) provides a useful resource for evaluating perception. Table 4–1 presents the areas in which a therapist evaluates a worker's perception.

Processing

Processing is the manner in which information is interpreted and in which decisions are based on this interpretation. Variables that affect processing include the worker's experience, education, emotions, and training. Table 4–2 presents the areas from the Standards of Practice useful in the evaluation of a worker's processing in the workplace.

Action

Action is the manner in which decisions are carried out. In the industrial setting, actions are completed through the use of tools. However, many tools require controls to operate. Examples of controls are handles, levels, computer keyboards, buttons, dials, and knobs. Table 4–3, adapted from the Standards of Practice, presents areas useful in the evaluation of action in a workplace.

TABLE 4–1 Perceptual Skills

Stereognosis	Identification of objects through the sense of touch.
Kinesthesia	Identification of the excursion and direction of joint movement.
Body Scheme	Acquisition of an internal awareness of the body and the relationship of body parts to each other.
Right-Left Discrimination	Differentiation of one side of the body from the other.
Form Consistency	Recognition of forms and objects as the same in various environments, positions, and sizes.
Position in Space	Determination of the spatial relationship of figures and objects to self or other forms and objects.
Visual Closure	Identification of forms or objects from incomplete presentation.
Figure Ground	Differentiation between foreground and background forms and objects.
Depth Perception	Determination of the relative distance between objects, figures, or landmarks.
Topographical Orientation	Determination of the location of objects and settings and the route to the location.

TABLE 4–2 Processing Performance Components

Sensory Motor Component	
Sensory Integration :	The combination of sensory awareness and sensory processing.
Sensory Awareness:	Reception of and differentiation of sensory stimuli.
Sensory Processing:	Interpretation of tactile, proprioceptive, vastibular, visual, and auditory sensory stimuli.
Tactile Processing:	Interpretation of light touch, pressure, temperature, pain, vibration, and two-point stimuli through skin contact/receptors.
Proprioceptive Processing:	Interpretation of stimuli that originate in muscles, joints, and other internal tissues to give information about the position of one body part in relation to another.
Vestibular Processing:	Interpretation of stimuli from inner ear reception regarding head position and movement.
Visual:	Interpretation of stimuli through the eyes, including peripheral vision and acuity, awareness of color, depth, and figure ground.
Auditory Processing:	Interpretation of stimuli through the ears.
Cognitive Integration and Cognitive Components	
Level of Arousal:	Demonstration of alertness and responsiveness to environmental stimuli.
Recognition:	Identification of familiar faces, objects, and other previously presented materials.
Attention Span:	Focus on a task over time.
Short-Term Memory:	Recall of information for brief periods of time.
Long-Term Memory:	Recall of information for long periods of time.
Remote Memory:	Recall of events from distant past.
Recent Memory:	Recall of events from immediate past.
Sequencing:	Placing information, concepts and actions in order.
Categorization:	Identification of similarities and differences in environmental information.

To use Tables 4–1, 4–2, and 4–3, the therapist conducts an activity analysis on a particular job to determine the areas most important for the successful completion of a task. After isolating these factors, the therapist systematically determines the areas that may lead to problems or risk for injury. A breakdown in cognitive workload can result in loss of productivity or in an injury. Tables 4–4 through 4–7 address the areas of perception, processing, and action. These tables are designed to be used in an industrial setting and are presented in a checklist format for easy use. Tables 4–4 and 4–5 assist the therapist in isolating the common problems seen in visual and auditory displays in industry. These tables are useful to therapists conducting

TABLE 4–3 Action

Neuromuscular	
Strength	Demonstration of a degree of muscle power when movement is resisted, as with weight or gravity.
Endurance	Sustained cardiac, pulmonary, and musculo-skeletal exertion over time.
Postural Control	Positioning and maintainance of head, neck, trunk, and limb alignment with appropriate weight shifting, midline orientation, and righting reactions for function.

Motor	
Activity Tolerance	Ability to sustain a purposeful activity over time.
Gross Motor Coordination	Use of large muscle groups for controlled movements.
Crossing the Midline	Movement of limbs and eyes across the sagittal plane of the body.
Laterality	Use of a preferred unilateral body part for activities requiring a high level of skill.
Bilateral Integration	Interaction between both sides of the body in a coordinated manner during activity.
Praxis	Conception and planning of a new motor act in response to an environmental demand.
Fine Motor Coordination/ Dexterity	Use of small muscle groups for controlled movements, particularly in object manipulation.
Visual-Motor Integration	Coordination of the interaction between visual information and body movement during activity.

on-site job analyses for clients in work-hardening programs and to therapists conducting ergonomic consultations for industry. When using these tables, it is important for the evaluator not only to observe the job tasks but also to interview the worker (Tables 4–4 and 4–5).

Table 4–6 presents a practical format that can be used by therapists performing job analyses or ergonomic consultations to determine processing problems in the industrial setting. In industry, the major concern is the speed and accuracy with which information is processed and transposed into action. When using Table 4–6, it is important for the therapist to remember that the worker is probably working under less than ideal circumstances and that extensive modification of the job will not be possible. Therefore, the therapist must use common sense when reviewing information-processing.

To design machines and systems for efficient action in the workplace, the designer must carefully evaluate the tools used to operate the system. Table 4–7 presents questions that a therapist can ask to determine if the tools are adequate for the task. Table 4–7 can be used by a therapist who is

TABLE 4–4 Evaluation of Visual Displays (Perception)

	Yes	No	Comments
Are displays clearly labeled?			
Are displays readable at required viewing distance?			
Are identifying marks easy to associate with designated controls?			
Are displays well lit?			
Does intensity of lighting have adverse effect on operation of controls?			
Does positioning of head and neck encourage good body mechanics when operator reads display?			
Is figure ground sufficient on dials, gauges, scales, and video screens?			
Are characters large enough to prevent eye strain?			
Can operator read dials accurately in time available?			
Are displays well organized with minimal scanning required?			
Are important displays located within line of sight and secondary displays located within 15° to 40° of viewing point?			
Is operator's field of vision within 15° around the line of sight for primary displays?			
Does operator verbalize difficulty with visual displays?			

Adapted from the UAW: Ford Ergonomics Process. UAW Ford National Joint Committee on Health and Safety, with permission.

conducting a job analysis for a client who is undergoing work hardening or a therapist who is conducting an ergonomic consultation.

Conclusion

To design ergonomically sound job tasks, the designer must consider cognitive workload, especially as it relates to information-processing. Observation is the best way to determine if cognitive workload is within acceptable limits. When evaluating cognitive workload, a therapist must evaluate whether or not all workers are having difficulty with a task. Because occupational therapists use activity as a treatment tool, knowledge of cognitive workload can be applied to many therapeutic situations. Because they have expertise

TABLE 4–5   Evaluation of Auditory Displays (Perception)

	Yes	No	Comments
Are auditory displays easily heard?			
Does background noise hamper signals from being heard accurately?			
Are similar signals easily differentiated?			
Are signals different enough from one another?			
Are there times when auditory signals are easier to differentiate than at others?			
Are there places in the work area where signals are easier to differentiate than in other places?			
Does pitch affect the operator's ability to differentiate signals?			
Does loudness affect the operator's ability to differentiate signals?			
Would a visual instead of an auditory signal enhance the operator's ability to distinguish signals?			
Would an auditory signal instead of a visual signal enhance the operator's ability to differentiate signals?			
Does operator speak in normal tones to be heard?			
Does operator have hearing loss in high or low ranges?			
Does operator verbalize difficulty with auditory display?			

Adapted from the UAW Ford Ergonomics Process. UAW Ford National Joint Committee on Health and Safety.

in areas that involve cognition, occupational therapists will find their practice enhanced by knowledge of cognitive workload.

References

Armstrong, T., Pannett, B., Ketner, P. (1984). Subjective worker assessment of hand tools used in automobile assembly. American Industrial Hygiene Association Journal, 50:639-645.

Borg, G. (1982). Psychophysical bases of perceived exertion. Medicine and Science in Sports and Exercise, 14:377-381.

Eysenck, H.J. (1962). Manual for the Eysenck Personality Inventory. San Diego: Education and Industrial Testing Service.

TABLE 4–6 Information Processing

	Yes	No	Comments
Is information presented too rapidly?			
Is Iinformation presented too slowly?			
Does operator rely on short-term memory to interpret and respond to data?			
Does operator rely on long-term memory to interpret and respond to data?			
Does operator require learning tools to assist with completion of task?			
Is operator training adequate to allow operator to make routine decisions about task?			
Does operator have difficulty with sequencing of task?			
Does operator have difficulty with sequencing at control panel?			
Is operator's attention to task disrupted by other tasks?			
Does operator handle emergencies according to policies and procedures?			
Does operator display difficulty with: concentration?			
With: decision making?			
With: problem solving?			
With: following directions?			
Is operator required to perform five steps in one procedure?			
Does operator verbalize difficulty in processing?			

Adapted from the UAW Ford Ergonomics Process. UAW Ford National Joint Committee on Health and Safety.

Fiori, N., Richardson, J., Boain, M. (1991). Operator workload and system performance under different conditions of force feedback in a telemanipulation task. Ergonomics, 34:193-210.

Frankenhaeser, M., Gardell, B. (1976). Underload and overload in working life: Outline of multidisciplinary approach. Journal of Human Stress, 2:35-46.

Frankenhaeser, M., Norhedon, B., Sjobert, H. (1969). Physiological and subjective reactions to different work loads. Perceptual Motor Skills, 28:343-349.

French, J., Calplan, R. (1972). Organization stress and individual strain. In A.J. Marrow (Ed.). The Failure of Success (pp. 30-66). Chicago: American Medical Association.

Friedman, M., Rosenman R. (1974). Type A behavior and your heart. New York: Alfred A. Knopf.

Gallagher, S. (1991). Acceptable weights and physiological costs of performing combined manual handling task in restricted postures. Ergonomics, 34:939-952.

Gamberale, F. (1988). Maximum acceptable workloads for repetitive lifting tasks: An experimental evaluation of psychophysical criteria. Presented at the Fourth

TABLE 4-7 Action

	Yes	No	Comments
Are controls grouped according to function?			
Are controls easily distinguished according to function?			
Are controls sequenced to reduce errors?			
Are emergency controls grouped together?			
Are emergency controls easily located?			
Is operator required to perform frequent movements above shoulder height?			
Is operator required to perform frequent repetitive movements at the control panel?			
Are color-coded controls easily understandable?			
Does operator verbalize difficulty with controls?			
Does operator correctly use touch controls?			
Are touch controls within comfortable reach?			
Is there figure-ground difficulty with controls?			
Are the controls designed to enhance stereognosis?			
Does protective equipment hamper operator's performance?			

Adapted from the UAW Ford Ergonomics Process. UAW Ford National Joint Committee on Health and Safety.

Finnish-U.S. Joint Symposium on Occupational Safety and Health, Turka, Finland, July 7-14, 1988.

Giannini, A.J., Daoud, J., Giannini, M.C., Boniface, R., Rhodes, P.G. (1978). Intellect versus intuition—A dichotomy in the reception of nonverbal communication. Journal of General Psychology, 99:19-23.

Gillet, M., Morgan, W. (1977). Influence of acute work activity on state anxiety. Journal of Psychosomatics, 15:179-181.

Gopher, D., Dauchin, E. (1986). Workload: An examination of the concept. In K. Boff, L. Kauffman, and J.P. Thomas (Eds.). Handbook of Perception and Human Performance (pp. 41-49). New York: Wiley.

Hart, S., Staveland, L. (1988). Development of the NASA task load index (TLX): Results of empirical and theoretical research. In P.A. Hancock and N. Meshkati (Eds.). Human Mental Workload (pp. 136-183). New York: Elsevier North Holland.

Hermansen, L., Saltin, B. (1956). Oxygen uptake during maximal work activity. Journal of Applied Physiology, 26:31-37.

Karase, R. (1979). Job demands, job decisions latitude and mental strain: Implications for job redesign. Administrative Science Quarterly, 24:285-308.

Kuronski, W. (1991). Psychophysical acceptability and perception of load heaviness in females. Ergonomics, 34:487-496.

Luce, R. (1972). What sort of measurement is psychophysical measurement? American Psychologist, 27:96-106.

Luczah, H. (1991). Work under extreme conditions. Ergonomics, 34:687-720.

Miller, R.E., Giannini, A.J., Levine, J.M. (1977). Nonverbal communication in man with a cooperative conditioning task. Journal of Social Psychology, 103:101-109.

Reid, G., Nygren, T. (1988). The subjective workload assessment technique: A scaling procedure for measuring mental workload. In P.A. Hancock and N. Meshkati (Eds.). Human Mental Workload (pp. 185-218). New York: Elsevier North Holland.

Rosenman, R. (1980). The relationship between type A behavior pattern to coronary heart disease. Activitus Nervosa Superior, 22:1-45.

Sanders, M., McCormick, E. (1987). Human Factors in Engineering and Design. New York: McGraw-Hill.

Shriver, D., Foto, M. (1983). Standards of Practice for Occupational Therapy. American Journal of Occupational Therapy, 37:802-804.

Stevens, S. (1962). The homeostatic and comfort perceptual systems. Journal of Psychology, 75:157-162.

Thurstone, O.L. (1951). The dimensions of temperament. Psychometrika, 16:11-20.

Tsang, P., Johnson, W. (1989). Cognitive demands in automation. Aviation Space and Environmental Medicine, 60:130-135.

Ulin, S.. Armstrong, T.O., Snook, S., Keyserling, W. (in press). Perceived exertion and discomfort associated with driving screws at various work locations and at different work frequencies. Ergonomics.

Ulin, S., Ways, C., Armstrong, T., Snook, S. (1990). Perceived exertion and discomfort versus work height with pistol shaped screwdriver. American Industrial Hygiene Association Journal, 51:528-594.

Wickens, C. (1984). Engineering Psychology and Human Performance. Columbus: Charles Merrill.

CHAPTER 5

Environmental Design

Peter Picone

ABSTRACT

Human factors practitioners evaluate the person, the environment, and the equipment in the design of a workplace. The perspective is a user-centered system design approach in which environmental variables are driving constraints. These variables include vibration, noise, illumination, and temperature. The human-engineering designer must compensate for each variable to arrive at a successful design.

In the field of human factors and ergonomics, all forms of system design, analysis, or review require that the therapist understand the concept that every task performed within a defined system is a function of the integration of three factors: the person performing the task, the equipment utilized, and the physical environment in which the operator and the equipment interact (Figure 5–1). The factors shown in the figure are inseparable for the purposes of design and analysis.

Many factors come into play in the description of the environment. The degree to which the factors affect performance depends on the harshness of the environment and the criticality of the tasks to be performed. For example, in the design of an airplane, considerations for the operational environment differ substantially for the pilot and the passenger. On the basis of criticality of the tasks to be performed and the physical and cognitive limitations of each operator, the physical design of the area around each is unique. In other

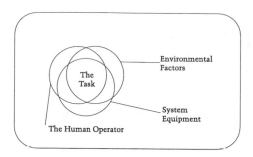

Figure 5–1   The performance environment.

words, the pilot is given a steering wheel and access to the throttles, but passengers have neither. The passenger has a tray table to hold food and drink, which the pilot should not need.

This chapter describes and quantifies a few of the constraints inherent in the operational environment and provides a perspective on designing for the benefit of the operator with those environmental constraints in mind. The environmental variables discussed include vibration, noise, illumination, and temperature. In each case, the definitions, terminology, and measurements are described, and the impact of each environmental variable on design is discussed.

Vibration

Vibration affects almost everyone regardless of his or her job or activity. In the workplace, vibration is felt most commonly in tasks that involve machinery and vehicles. It can take the form of whole-body vibration, usually transmitted to the person through a vehicle seat or the shop floor, or it can be transmitted in a segmental manner and isolated locally, such as arm and hand vibration in the use of a hand tool, such as a drill, a grinder, or a saw. Vibration can be of low or high frequency, of a wide variety of intensities, and can occur in combinations of single frequencies and resonant harmonic frequencies.

Definitions, Terms, and Measurements

Mechanical vibration can be measured and described mathematically in terms of both frequency and time domains. These measurements include Fourier analysis, modal analysis, transfer function analysis, and mechanical impedance analysis, to name a few. The details of these methods can be found in a good mechanical engineering text, such as Cannon's *Dynamics of Physical Systems* (Cannon, 1967). The terms and physical concepts impor-

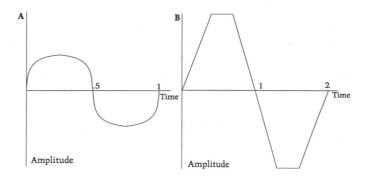

Figure 5–2   Frequency of a vibration.

tant in the discussion and understanding of the effects of vibration on the body are as follows.

Frequency

The frequency of a sound or vibration is the number of complete cycles per second made by a vibration. In Figure 5–2, vibration A completes one full cycle per second. Its frequency is 1 hertz (Hz). Vibration B completes only half of its cycle in 1 second; therefore, its frequency is 0.5 Hz.

Amplitude

The amplitude of a vibration is represented by the amount of movement from a mean position to the extreme. It is a measurement of the power of the vibration. In Figure 5–2, if the units of the amplitude scale are the same for vibration A and for vibration B, vibration B has a greater amplitude than vibration A.

Form factor

Form factor is the differentiation in shape of a vibration. In Figure 5–2, vibration A has a smooth form and vibration B, a jagged form. If these vibrations were musical tones, the clean sinusoidal shape of vibration A would sound like a note from a flute or a guitar string, whereas vibration B would sound like a harmonica.

Resonance

Resonance is the vibrating frequency at which maximum mechanical energy is transferred from the vibrating source to a person. At resonance, the person is maximally "tuned" to the vibrating source, and the vibrational movement of the human tissue (when properly synchronized) amplifies the power of the vibrating source.

Harmonics

A harmonic vibration is a periodic vibration the frequency of which is an integral multiple of the fundamental or base frequency. For example, if the fundamental frequency is 50 Hz, the first harmonic is 100 Hz, the second harmonic is 150 Hz, the third harmonic is 200 Hz, and so on.

Differentiation Between Noise and Whole-Body Accelerations

Vibration can affect the human body in many ways. Air-borne vibration striking the ear causes the eardrum to vibrate in resonance with the incoming changes in air pressure, and the vibration is perceived as sound. Mechanical vibration of different frequencies interacts with the human body, and parts of the body respond by vibrating in resonance with the external vibration. This resonance effect often amplifies the incoming vibration and can damage the part of the body in resonance. This section discusses the mechanical transmission of vibration to the body and the effects of this transmission. The section on noise examines the effect of vibration on the ear and the consideration of this effect in the design process. Additional references for exposure limits and recommended tolerances can be found in the *Guide for Evaluation of Human Exposure to Whole-Body Vibration* compiled by the International Organization for Standardization (1974).

Different parts of the body resonate at different frequencies. In the vertical direction, the whole body (mostly the torso) resonates in the range of 4 to 8 Hz (usually at 5 Hz). In the horizontal and lateral directions, resonance is in the range of 1 to 2 Hz (Coermann, 1962). The head and shoulders tend to resonate at 10 to 20, and the eyeballs resonate at 60 to 80 Hz (Grether, 1971).

The effects of vibration on performance are difficult to quantify. Different frequencies affect different parts of the body in different ways. Frequencies fall into three general categories: (1) general discomfort, (2) disruption of visual acuity, and (3) at frequencies greater than 100 Hz, a tickling sensation in the hands and feet. General discomfort has negative motivational and physiologic effects on operator performance. Disruptions in visual performance can result in degradation of any task that requires eye-hand coordination, especially tasks in which reading and writing are important. Loss of visual acuity can become extremely hazardous in some occupations. For example, a helicopter pilot with a vibration-induced lack of visual acuity may not see electrical high-tension wires.

The severity of the tickling sensation in the hands and feet is related to the duration and intensity of the vibration. When intensity is high and duration is long, as in the case of chain-saw operators, physiologic damage can occur. The threshold for this type of damage is approximately 1g at 100

Hz, and the rise thereafter is 6 decibels (dB) per octave (May, 1978). At lower intensities and shorter durations, fine manipulative skills can be disrupted; the extreme case is the development of "dead hands" (Raynaud phenomenon of occupational origin, vibrational white fingers). In its early stages, this syndrome causes occasional tingling, numbness, and blanching of the fingers. With repeated exposure, the disease acquires a peripheral vascular component (intermittent blanching and cyanosis of all fingertips except the thumb) episodes of which last 15 to 30 minutes. In its most extreme form, the disease progresses to gangrene of the affected fingers. Cold temperatures tend to trigger the attacks, and both fevers and smoking exacerbate the problem (Salvendy, 1987).

Noise

Although sound is simply exposure to oscillating vibrations in the form of pressure changes at the ear, the impact of sound on a human operator and general performance can be quite different from that of other mechanical vibrations. Confronting noise in a work environment involves examination of the system from two perspectives: the direct physical attributes of noise and vibration and the subjective responses to those physical attributes. Each of these perspectives influences the design approach.

Definitions, Terms, and Measurements

Sound pressure level

The sound pressure level (SPL) of the energy that impinges on the ear is measured in decibels (dB). In mathematical terms, it is defined as follows

$$SPL = 20 \log_{10} \frac{P_n}{P_{ref}}$$

where P_n is the root mean square sound pressure produced by the source being measured and P_{ref} is a standard reference value that corresponds roughly to the minimum pressure detectable by the human ear, usually considered to be 20 micropascals (2×10^{-5} Pa = 2×10^{-5} N/m^2 = 2×10^4 μbar). Thus, the SPL is an absolute ratio of two pressure magnitudes with respect to the minimum audible SPL (International Labor Office, 1980). This is an excellent physical measurement, but because the human ear does not perceive sound equally across the entire range of audible frequencies, the definition is often modified to include tailoring for the frequency biases of the ear. Modifying the weighting in some of the frequency bands results in a sound level that to some extent correlates with the loudness of a sound as heard by the listener. These weighted scales dB(A) and dB(C) are used to measure the "loudness" of a sound as opposed to its direct pressure ratio. This modification allows one to evaluate sound or noise in an environment on the basis of the way it is perceived by the human ear and then how the person responds.

Loudness, noisiness, and annoyance

Loudness is defined as the subjective magnitude of a sound. This refers only to how intensely the sound is perceived, not to how the listener evaluates its content. The "unwantedness" of the sound, as it is sometimes known, should not be considered loudness. The degree to which a sound is considered "noisy" is defined as the degree of unwantedness of the sound and is considered separately from loudness. Finally, the noisiness of a sound results in an associated degree of "annoyance." Annoyance is defined as the overall unwantedness of a sound heard in a natural situation. A person's judgment of the annoyance of a sound includes the degree of "noisiness" inherent in the sound and many other variables related to the context in which the sound is heard (Peterson & Gross, 1978). A sound heard during the night can be much more annoying than the same sound heard during the day. Anyone who has ever lain in bed listening to a dripping faucet or running toilet knows of this phenomenon. Likewise, a repeated sound may be more annoying when a worker is attempting to concentrate on a task than if it were encountered when the worker was more relaxed. That same sound can become even more annoying when the listener is unable to remove the sound. When they have the option of turning off an auditory warning, machine operators consider the sound less objectionable than if they were forced to listen to it until a supervisor turned off the alarm.

Speech interference and intelligibility

Speech interference is a function of the loudness of a sound, not simply its SPL. Measurements of interference and intelligibility are generally based on a calculation of the percentage of words, phrases, or sentences correctly understood over a specific speech communication system in a particular noise environment. This can pertain to both human-to-human communication and to human-to-machine speech recognition systems (Picone, 1983). Interference and intelligibility are typically measured using either the Phonetically Balanced Monosyllabic Word Intelligibility Test or the Modified Rhyme Test. In the former test a list of 1000 words is dictated by a source (usually a tape recording), and the listener responds by crossing off or marking a word on a preformatted list of options. In the Modified Rhyme Test a source reads aloud a list of 300 words, and a listener selects from a prepared multiple-word formatted list one of six words as the word heard for each spoken word. For example, the speaker says, "Would you please circle the word *gold* now." The listener then selects the word from a six-word choice grouping that consists of the words *mold, bold, sold, gold, hold,* and *cold.*

Speech intelligibility also may be predicted by use of the articulation index. In this index the peak speech-to-root mean square noise ratio is calculated in selected frequency bands. The bands used range from 200 to 7000 Hz (the range of frequencies that contain the most information with regard to speech content). The articulation index is a measurement of the peak amplitude of speech in relation to the "average" amplitude of the background noise. In each of these cases, what is being measured is the degree to which a sound that contains information necessary for the interpretation of that sound as speech is being masked by ambient background noise. In the case of the two phonetic lists, one directly measures the degradation that has occurred in a communication system (even if the system is in an open-air, face-to-face environment). In the case of the articulation index, one takes a predictive measurement of the anticipated decrement in speech performance based on the amount of meaningful sound energy available over the background clutter.

Auditory Effects of Noise

Audible frequencies

The human auditory system has an extremely wide range of sensitivity to the spectrum of sound amplitude. This drives the measurement of sound intensity to a logarithmic scale (the decibel) to cover the entire range. Human sensitivity to the frequency of sound is much less than the sensitivity to amplitude. The full range of frequencies perceivable by a human roughly covers the bands from 20 Hz on the low end to 20,000 Hz on the high end. This range varies widely with factors such as age or hearing loss due to physical damage to the auditory system (Woodson, 1981).

Hazardous noise limitations

Two types of sound must be considered in the assessment of noise hazards—continuous noise and impact noise. Continuous noises are what people most commonly encounter. These are repetitive sounds of a slowly fluctuating intensity that have relatively slow rise and fall times. Examples include a noisy street or the background noise in an office. Impact noise is a sound with an almost instantaneous rise and fall time; it usually reaches a very high intensity for a very short time. Examples include gunshots, cars backfiring, or noises made by some factory machines, such as automated looms or presses.

Hazardous properties of noise

Concepts to be kept in mind in the evaluation of hazardous noise are as follows:

- Low-frequency noise energy tends to be less damaging to hearing than middle-frequency noise
- Damage to a particular frequency band is caused by a sound an octave below that region. For example, exposure to intense sound at a frequency of 8000 Hz causes damage to the listener's sensitivity at 16,000 Hz.
- Susceptibility to noise-induced hearing losses varies from person to person.
- Beyond certain levels, high sound intensity and long exposure time produce extensive hearing losses, and a large percentage of the people in the group exposed have an extensive hearing loss.
- Hearing loss due to noise is most pronounced at about 4000 Hz but spreads over the frequency range as exposure time and level increase.

Over the years, studies have isolated properties of noise exposure that contribute most heavily to the destruction of the neurologic elements of the ear and to consequent hearing loss. Of these properties, the most critical are the overall noise level, the spectrum of the noise, the total duration of exposure, and the temporal distribution of the noise.

Noise Level.   It is usually safe to assume that a noise level less than 80 dB(A), although potentially annoying, will not cause any temporary or permanent hearing damage. In the presence of a noise level greater than 80 dB(A), it is necessary to assess other criteria before defining the noise as hazardous.

Noise Spectrum.   The noise spectrum is the range of component frequencies of the noise. As mentioned earlier, the frequency at which damage occurs in the presence of excessive SPLs depends on the frequencies of the noise causing the damage. A single noise may have many different component frequencies, and each of those frequencies may be present at a different level of intensity. If one of the components is of a damaging magnitude, then damage will most likely occur relative to that frequency rather than to any of the others.

Duration of Exposure.   Brief exposure to relatively loud SPLs, regardless of the frequency of the sound, may be tolerated without long-term damage. The most hazardous exposure is one in which continuous exposure occurs throughout a full period of work (eg, an 8-hour day). The Department of Labor has adopted a recommended allowable exposure level (Table 5–1). The allowance begins at 90 dB(A) for an 8-hour day.

Temporal Distribution.   Temporal distribution is exposure to a sound over time in which the exposure is not uniform. For example, airport ground crews are exposed to very loud jet engine noises (115 to 125 dB[A]) for very short periods of time (2 to 3 minutes) every time a plane pulls in or takes off from

Table 5–1   Allowable Noise Exposures

Duration (Hours/Day)	Sound Level (dB[A])	Example
8	90	Subway car at 20 ft.
6	92	
4	95	
3	97	
2	100	Punch press at 3 ft.
1.5	102	
1	105	
0.25 or less	115	Jet engine noise

the gate. Although this noise falls well within the exposure guidelines, there is still a strong possibility that it may prove damaging in the long term. Because of this risk, the crew should always wear hearing protection.

Exposure and Frequency Relationships

It is always prudent to keep hazardous and unwanted noise and vibration levels in the workplace below the recommended maximum levels. For best results, efforts to remove or isolate unwanted noise and vibration can only benefit a design. When it is not possible to redesign the environment, steps should be taken to redesign the task so as to reduce exposure time, to use personal protective hearing devices whenever possible, or to use a combination of both measures.

When the opportunity to redesign the work environment does exist, methods of control include reduction of a noise or vibration at its source and prevention of propagation, amplification, or reverberation of the noise. Methods typically involve the use of acoustic or mechanical damping devices. Often minor changes can control auditory environments. For example, a room can be altered by changing the density of a carpet, adding acoustic tile to a ceiling, using screens or soundproof partitions, or hanging acoustic damping materials on walls. Vibration can often be controlled by mounting vibrating equipment on damping platforms to isolate the equipment from the floor or by providing noise-isolating enclosures for the equipment.

When it is not possible to alter the environment, workers should wear hearing protection, and the type of protection used should be considered carefully. The protection should not interfere with the tasks to be performed and should be compatible with the equipment the operator uses. For example, safety glasses may interfere with the effectiveness of earmuff-type protective devices because the temple piece of the glasses may break the seal at the ear. General hygiene factors also should be considered. Each worker should have his or her own hearing-protection device, especially if earplugs are used.

When possible, disposable ear protection is preferred over reusable devices. Additional care should be given to training the worker on the proper use of the device. For example, foam inserts lose a major percentage of their effectiveness when the incorrect size is used or when they are improperly inserted into the ear canal. Finally, providing workers with hearing-protection devices does does not ensure they will use them. Workers should be regularly encouraged to use the devices provided to protect their hearing.

Use of Auditory Displays

Audio displays are typically used when the information to be provided is short, simple, and transitory in nature and requires an immediate response. Typically these responses are used to warn, alert, or cue an operator that a response is required (Military Standard, 1989). Audio displays fall into two categories: verbal and nonverbal. A verbal audio display usually is preceded by a nonverbal tone to attract the operator's attention. A well-known example of this type of display is used in automobiles in which a tone sounds and a synthesized voice immediately states: "Your door is ajar." Nonverbal displays are either pure periodic tones such as the beep a computer makes or more complex sounds such as doorbell chimes. Design considerations for both verbal and nonverbal displays include the following:

1. The frequency range used
2. How frequently the signal occurs
3. The intensity of the signal
4. The compatibility of the signal with the acoustic environment
5. The compatibility of the signal with operator constraints or limitations (eg, whether or not the operator wears hearing protection or a protective mask or headgear)
6. The ease of discernment between the signal and other auditory displays in use
7. The onset and SPL of the signal and the distance over which the signal must be heard
8. If headsets are used, to which ear the signal is presented

Illumination and Lighting

In its purest form, detailed lighting and illumination design is an art best left to specialists in the field. This chapter discusses the concepts required for a designer to make a basic assessment of the lighting in a work situation. There is also a brief discussion of the relation between lighting factors and operation of a video display terminal (VDT).

Definitions, Terms, and Measurements

The Illuminating Engineering Society (IES) Lighting Handbook (Kaufman & Haynes, 1984) begins with a 40-page dictionary of lighting terminology essential for practicing lighting engineers. The reader should study this source before attempting any lighting design or redesign project.

Light can be defined as any radiant energy capable of exciting the human retina and producing a visual sensation. In physics, visible light is regarded as that portion of the electromagnetic spectrum that lies between the wavelengths 380 to 770 nm. However, as with the auditory system, these upper and lower limits of wavelength vary from person to person. Radiant energy in this band of the electromagnetic spectrum makes visible anything from which it is emitted or reflected in sufficient quantity to activate the receptors of the eye (Kaufman & Haynes, 1984). Responses from the receptors of the eyes are then interpreted by the brain as visual perception. Associated with this perception are all of the perceptual and psychologic foibles to which the brain is often subject. Radiant energy is measured in a number of ways. Two of the most common are radiant flux and luminous flux.

Radiant flux

Radiant flux is the rate of flow of radiant energy. It is usually expressed in watts or joules per second. Light-bulb strength is measured in watts, or the amount of radiant energy given off in a certain time period.

Luminous flux

Luminous flux is the time rate of flow of light. In the Système International (SI) measurement system, it is measured in lumens. A light bulb is often rated in terms of the average number of lumens as well as the wattage. The radiometric evaluation of luminous flux is based on the amount of radiant power. The photometric evaluation is based on the luminous flux emitted within a unit solid angle (1 steradian) by a point source that has a uniform luminous intensity of 1 candela. A candela is the SI measurement of luminous intensity. One candela is equal to 1 lumen per steradian. A much more specific definition entails the wavelength of the light and the power density of the light.

The following definitions specify what happens to light energy once it has been generated by its source:

Reflectance

Reflectance is the amount of incident light not transmitted or absorbed by a surface. It is usually described as the ratio of reflected light to incident light.

Transmittance

Transmittance is the amount of light that passes through a surface or a body. When struck by light, a pane of glass reflects some light and allows some light to pass through. The amount of light that passes through is described by the transmittance level.

Absorption

Absorption is the amount of light not transmitted or reflected by a surface. It is the general term for the process by which incident light is converted into another form of energy, usually heat. One can see an example of this phenomenon merely by putting one's hand next to a light bulb and feeling the incident light turning to heat as it is absorbed by the hand.

Glare

Glare is the sensation produced by light in a visual field that is considerably brighter than the light level to which the eyes are accustomed. Glare usually results in annoyance, discomfort, and loss of visual performance or visibility.

General Lighting Design Techniques

There are two general approaches to lighting design: designing in relation to the luminous environment and designing in relation to the visual task. They are fully compatible, and both should be considered in any evaluation.

General guidelines

Consideration of Spatial Function.   Lighting must conform to the activity. In a warehouse, the activity may be driving a forklift and reading package labeling. In a law office, it may be reading fine print in a contract. Both may require different lighting levels and coloration.

Provision of Quality and Quantity of Illumination.   The designer must consider the visual sense and how a person perceives the visual environment. The designer must consider not only where a task is performed but also how the periphery is perceived. For example, one must determine how many lights are needed, how they should be shielded, and whether they will produce annoying glare on a surface.

Selection of the Lighting Systems, Lighting Sources, and Luminaires.   A therapist involved in the redesign of an environment should consider not only the engineering specifications of how much lighting is required and where it should be placed but also whether the lighting should be local, general, supplemental, or task-ambient in nature and whether the quality of the fixture should be direct, indirect, diffuse, or a combination of these qualities.

The designer also must recognize environmental constraints, such as the amount of dust or dirt in the area and how color balancing will influence the task or the perception of space.

Selection of the Lighting Control Systems.   The designer must determine if the lighting should be controlled in groups of lights or individually; where controls should be located in relation to traffic flow; and if the controls should be discrete (on-off switch) or continuously dimmable.

Consideration of Economics.   The designer must consider the client's budget. For example, a solid brass fixture on a gold chain may complement marble floors, but less expensive recessed-can lighting may perform just as well.

Coordination with Mechanical and Acoustical Systems.   The design of one system cannot be separated from that of the entire environment. Often, the ideal place for a lighting fixture is already occupied by an air-conditioning duct or sound barriers. Likewise, the location of a built-in fixture could force the relocation of a workstation and the disruption of an entire floor plan. All systems and the operational environment should be coordinated in the planning phase.

Coordination with Furniture.   In many work environments, the general ceiling lighting can serve primarily as supplemental lighting, and the critical fixtures can be built into the workstation furniture. The built-in fixtures can serve as direct task lighting, or they can throw diffuse lighting toward the ceiling to obviate the need for other free-standing fixtures.

Luminous environment design approach

Three steps are considered in the analysis.

Step 1.   Determine the Visual Composition of the Space

1. Focal centers
2. The overhead zone
3. The perimeter zone
4. The occupied zone
5. Transitional considerations
6. Levels of sensory stimulation

Step 2.   Determine the Desired Appearance of Objects in Space

1. Diffusion
2. Sparkle
3. Color rendition

Step 3.   Select Lighting to Accomplish Steps 1 and 2

1. The engineering study
    *   Distribution characteristics and coloration of light
    *   Dimensional characteristics and form
    *   Lighted and unlighted appearance of other materials
    *   Initial and operating costs
    *   Maintenance
    *   Energy consumption
2. The architectural study
    *   Brightness, color, scale, and form
    *   Compatibility with the period of the design
    *   Space requirements and architectural detailing
    *   Coordination with other environmental systems
3. The architectural context of the lighting
    *   Visually subordinate lighting systems
    *   Visually prominent lighting systems

Visual-task–oriented design approach

The general design is the same as for the luminous environment design approach, but the focus is on enhancing the task to be performed rather than on overall aesthetics of the situation. The steps are as follows:

Step 1.   Analyze the Visual Task

1. Determine the commonly found visual tasks performed in the environment
2. Determine how the task should be portrayed by the lighting
    *   Diffuse or directional
    *   Importance of shadows to provide a three-dimensional effect
    *   Susceptibility of task to veiling reflections
    *   Importance of coloration of the lighting
3. Determine illuminances to be provided

Step 2.   Analyze the Area in which the Task Is Performed

1. Measure the dimensions of the area and determine the reflective qualities of the surfaces
2. Determine the surface luminance required to minimize transition adaptation effects without providing a bland environment
3. Determine whether the surfaces produce unwanted glare
4. Determine whether uniformity in illumination is desirable

Step 3.   Select Light Fixtures

1. Determine the type of distribution, control mechanism, and spectral quality needed to perform the task and provide a visually comfortable environment
2. Determine the type of fixture needed to illuminate the work surfaces
3. Decide how the lighting fixture should look and how it should be mounted
4. Determine the atmosphere of the area and therefore the maintenance requirements, because dusty, dirty, and greasy environments put specific demands on the type of fixture used and determine how often they will need to be cleaned or replaced
5. Determine the cost of the lighting system in relation to the budget

Step 4.   Calculate, Lay Out, and Evaluate

1. Arrange the lighting fixtures to best portray the task. Consider illuminance, direction of illumination, veiling reflections, and disabling glare
2. Arrange fixtures to provide the most comfortable situation for the worker. Consider visual and thermal effects and direct and reflected glare. Mobility and traffic patterns may also be factors here
3. Provide an aesthetically pleasing arrangement
4. Determine the energy-management requirements

Each of the two approaches has its merits. Regardless of the background of the analyst—architect or ergonomist—each approach should produce similar results when applied to most industrial or commercial environments. In most cases, both perspectives should be examined.

Light and the Use of Visual Display Terminals

Some workers have tasks and functions that are so specific general guidelines not only do not suffice but also may do more harm than good. One such environment that has received much attention is the computer workstation. More than 50 million Americans use VDTs on a regular basis. Many of them often experience difficulty focusing on distant objects, a general blurring of vision beyond close range, eyestrain, irritated eyes, headaches, and intermittent blurring of images on the screen.

The two most common of these problems are breakdowns of eye focus and abnormalities in eye coordination. In addition to physical symptoms, problems related to the visual stress of the task include posture-related changes such as neck, shoulder, and back pain; frequent loss of place while trying to concentrate on work tasks; and excessive fatigue and irritability (Godnig & Hacunda, 1991).

Two types of problems are associated with use of a VDT. The first is hardware-related, and the second is software-related. In some situations the areas overlap. For example, the colors on the screen are generated by the hardware, but the specifications for the color are generated by a programmer in the software. Beyond the physical problems of neck and back strain, psychologic, perceptual and other performance-related problems can be traced to either of these sources. For example, a common perceptual problem in the use of VDTs is color shifts. After an operator views a source of light, such as a VDT, for some time, an afterimage of the display remains in the user's vision. This is similar to but not as severe as the spot that remains in front of the subject's eyes after a photograph is taken with a flash camera. In the case of a VDT, the afterimage takes on the opposite color of that being looked at. For example, after one uses a green screen, a pinkish glow persists for some time. Although this afterimage is harmless and dissipates in time, effects such as these may become important if supplemental tasks require the recognition of color-coded warnings.

Another perceptual problem that affects human performance during use of a VDT is polarity. Polarity relates to the use of black letters on a bright screen or bright letters on a black screen. The most common configuration is bright letters on a black screen. However, for tasks such as word processing, the foreground-to-background contrast provided by reverse polarity (black letters on a bright screen) and the similarity of this presentation style to that of print on paper makes text more readable than when conventional polarity is used. To eliminate the potential impact of eye fatigue when using a monochrome cathode ray tube (CRT), the user should be given the option of reversing the polarity at will to fit the task at hand.

A hardware-related problem that affects user performance is the luminance and contrast ratios of the screen and the interaction with the operating environment. Most monitors allow the user to adjust the brightness and contrast levels of the display. The user should be able to adjust the monitor to best perform in the ambient light. A standard for evaluating these limits is the 10-3-1 rule. That is, the contrast ratio between the text on the screen and its background should be 10:1 (text ten times brighter than the background). The overall brightness of the ambient environment should be three times brighter than the screen background (Godnig & Hacunda, 1991).

There are many other guidelines associated with hardware in the design and use of VDTs as well as with general workstation design. The role of graphic user interfaces and new software designs are influencing the requirements to use pointing devices such as mice, trackballs, pen interfaces, and thumb balls. An entire field of design is developing for both hardware and software (ANSI-STD-800-1, 1987).

Temperature

To remain alive, human beings must be able to regulate the internal temperature of their bodies to keep them within a small range of temperatures. This
balance is maintained by taking in, retaining, or putting out heat from the
body under the control of either the body itself or the environment. The
heat-balance equation states that the body's metabolic heat production must
equal its heat dissipation. Dissipation can take the form of evaporation,
radiation, conduction, or convection. All these methods of dissipation depend
on the internal and external environments of the body, and none can be fully
defined without some reference to either environment.

Definitions, Terms, and Measurements

Evaporation

The rate of evaporation of liquid from a surface is expressed as the volume of
liquid evaporated from a unit area of that surface in a unit measure of time.
A sample evaporation rate is 2 cubic centimeters of water per minute per
square inch of skin. Critical environmental factors involved in evaporation
include the surface wind speed, the temperatures of both the air and the
surface, the physical nature of the surface (the type of material), the amount
of liquid at the surface available for evaporation, and the relative humidity
of the air. The process of evaporation can be broken into two stages. The first
is the conduction of fluid to the evaporative surface. The second is the
removal of the newly formed vapor by surface air currents. The first stage is
perspiration; the second is convection and is related to wind speed.

Temperature

Temperature is a measurement of heat energy. It is also a measurement of
the ability of one body to transfer heat to or receive heat from another body.
In a two-body system, the body that looses heat to another body is considered
to have the higher temperature. In environmental design, one body is the
human operator in a system and the other is the mass of air that surrounds
the operator. In this context, there is a continuous exchange of heat between
the two bodies. Temperature is measured with a thermometer in degrees
Celsius, Fahrenheit, or Kelvin. Two types of liquid-in-glass thermometers are
commonly used for measuring temperature: dry-bulb and wet-bulb thermometers. Dry-bulb thermometers are conventional thermometers with
which most people are familiar. A wet-bulb thermometer is a dry-bulb
thermometer the bulb of which is surrounded by a water-soaked muslin wick.

The wet-bulb measurement allows for the evaporative quality of the air. As water evaporates from the wick, it takes with it the latent heat from the bulb. This cools the bulb and lowers the measured temperature by an amount that depends on the humidity of the surrounding air. The difference between the wet-bulb and dry-bulb temperatures is used to determine the relative humidity of the air.

Wet bulb globe temperature

One of the methods of heat exchange is radiation. A body as it receives heat energy from another body (such as the sun or a hot industrial furnace) begins to radiate its own energy. According to the Stephan Boltzman law, radiant heat energy is a function of the gradient between the two temperatures raised to the fourth power. This law also applies to "black bodies"—those that radiate the maximum amount for a given temperature. For evaluating the radiative heat environment, a third type of thermometer, the black globe thermometer, is used to measure the globe temperature. This thermometer is placed inside a black copper globe and placed adjacent to the wet- and dry-bulb thermometers.

The wet-bulb globe temperature (WBGT) index is used as the parameter to determine the environmental conditions for implementation of work practices. It is calculated using the following equations:

Indoor exposure or outdoor exposure with no solar load

$$WBGT = 0.7\,WB + 0.3\,GT$$

Outdoor sunlit exposure with solar load

$$WBGT = 0.7WB + 0.2GT + 0.1DB,$$

where WB is the wet-bulb temperature obtained with a wetted sensor exposed to the natural air movement (unaspirated); GT is the globe temperature measured at the interior of a 6-inch black globe; and DB is the dry-bulb temperature (U.S. Department of Health Education and Welfare, 1972).

Effective temperature

Effective temperature is an arbitrary index that combines in a single value the effects of temperature, humidity, and air movement on the sensation of warmth or cold felt by the human body. The numerical value is that of the temperature of still, saturated air, which would induce an identical sensation.

Thermal comfort

Thermal comfort is a function of both the effective temperature and the person's degree of acclimation to the particular environment.

Acclimation

Acclimation is the adaptive process of the body that results in the reduction of severity of the body's reactions to the stresses of exceptionally high or low temperatures. When a body is first exposed to a hot environment, the person has an impaired ability to work and evidence of physiologic strain. If the exposure is repeated over a period of several days, the ability to work returns, and the evidence of physiologic strain decreases. Within the first 4 to 7 days after initial exposure, there is a dramatic improvement in the ability to work, and physiologic responses such as body temperature and average heart rate decrease, blood pressure becomes stable, the subjective reaction of discomfort is reduced, and sweat is profuse and diluted. In general, a person who is in good physical condition acclimates fairly quickly, and an obese or overweight person finds it difficult to adapt.

Design for Hot Environments

Designing for a hot environment requires consideration of the level of acclimation of the operators and the psychologic effects of exposure to heat. Even a fully acclimated person who shows no decreased ability to perform physical work in a hot environment may still be sensitive to the heat and may show a decreased psychologic capability. These psychologic factors include a loss of mental initiative, a decrease in accuracy of work performed (especially for operators who were poorly motivated to begin with), the need for greater concentration to perform a task, and the possibility of general personality changes (including irritability and a shortened temper). Care should be taken to investigate fully the physical barriers imposed by an extremely hot environment. These include protective gloves, which reduce an operator's ability to perform fine manipulative tasks and necessitate that equipment controls be farther apart than usual to allow for operation by a gloved hand, and protective masks, which may reduce visibility and hearing and increase the effects of the heat.

Design for Cold Environments

When an operator's surroundings are exceptionally cold, the body must increase its metabolic output to maintain the heat-balance equation and must alter its internal blood distribution to protect the vital organs. The body begins to shiver and experience pain and numbness and reduced blood flow to the extremities, which causes a severe reduction in the ability to perform fine manipulative tasks. As with a hot environment, care should be taken to ensure that a system operator in a cold environment is fully acclimated before he or she assumes responsibility for any task. Additional clothing restricts the operator in much the same way as protection in a hot environment. In addition, operators in a cold environment may experience a lack of mobility if excessive clothing is required.

Conclusion

In the field of ergonomics, it is important to assimilate a general knowledge of many diverse topics into a holistic design approach and solution. Most of the time the designer finds that no matter how well he or she knows a topic, additional research is required to apply specific principles to a new problem. The following references should provide insight into ergonomic design principles involved in designing for a specific environment. The designer must remember, however, that the environment is only one of the three factors that should be considered before a design is complete. Ignoring the role of the operator or of the equipment can be just as hazardous as ignoring the role of the environment and its eventual impact on the success or failure of a design solution.

References

ANSI-STD-800-1 (1987). Human Factor Standards for VDT Workstations. American National Standards Institute. U.S. Government.

Cannon, R.H., Jr. (1967). Dynamics of Physical Systems. New York: McGraw-Hill.

Coermann, R.R. (1962). The mechanical impedance of the human body in sitting and standing positions at low frequencies. Human Factors, 4:225-253.

Godnig, E.C., Hacunda, J.S. (1991). Computers and Visual Stress: Staying Healthy. Grand Rapids, Mich.: Abacus.

Grether, W.F. (1971). Vibration and human performance. Human Factors, 13:203-205.

International Labor Office (1980). Protection of Workers Against Noise and Vibration in the Working Environment. ILO Codes of Practice. Geneva: International Labor Office.

International Organization for Standardization (1974). Guide for the Evaluation of Human Exposure to Whole-body Vibration. Report No. ISO 2631. International Organization for Standardization.

Kaufman, J.E., Haynes, H. (Eds.) (1982). Illuminating Engineering Society Lighting Handbook: Application. Baltimore: Waverly.

Kaufman, J.E., Haynes, H. (Eds.) (1984). Illuminating Engineering Society Lighting Handbook: Reference. Baltimore: Waverly.

May, D.N. (1978). Handbook of Noise Assessment. Van Nostrand Reinhold Environmental Engineering Series. New York: Van Nostrand Reinhold.

Military Standard: Human Engineering Design Criteria for Military Systems, Equipment and Facilities (1989). MIL-STD-1472D. U.S. Government.

Peterson, A.P.G., Gross, E.E. (1978). Handbook of Noise Measurement. Concord, Mass.: GENRAD.

Picone, P. (1983). Learning Systems and Pattern Recognition in Industrial Control. Proceedings of the 9th Annual Advanced Controls Conference, Purdue University, Sept. 21-23, 1983. Kompass, E.J., Williams, T.J. (Eds.) Barrington, Ill.: Technical Publishing, Dunn & Bradstreet.

Salvendy, G. (1987). Handbook of Human Factors (pp. 650-669). New York: Wiley.

U.S. Department of Health, Education, and Welfare (1972). Criteria for a Recommended Standard: Occupational Exposure to Hot Environments. Washington, D.C.: US Government Printing Office.

Woodson, W.E. (1981). Human Factors Design Handbook: Information and Guidelines for the Design of Systems, Facilities, Equipment, and Products for Human Use. New York: McGraw-Hill.

CHAPTER 6

Human Factors in Medical Rehabilitation Equipment: Product Development and Usability Testing

Valerie J. Berg Rice

ABSTRACT

The development of an assistive walker is used to illustrate usability testing (user-acceptance testing) and to describe the usability-testing process. Product development has three phases: initial development, efficacy testing, and comparison testing. The three phases are equivalent to pilot, laboratory, and field testing. These phases help to ensure that the final product docs what it was designed to do, is acceptable to the people who use it, and is easy to use. Each of these phases of product development has a nine-step testing process. The philosophy of usability testing is to match the product with human capabilities, limitations, and acceptance, producing an environment or product that is user-friendly.

Two groups who use medical and rehabilitation equipment are medical personnel and clients. Therefore, equipment should be evaluated for effectiveness, ease of use, comfort, and acceptability for both populations. This evaluation process is referred to as usability testing. Usability testing (also referred to as evaluative testing or development research) is most effective when performed throughout the product-development process. However, it can be accomplished during any or all of the stages of product development (Meister, 1989). Usability testing provides valuable information for equipment design, recommendation, and purchase. This chapter describes the product-development and usability-testing process. Development of a walker is used as an example.

Overview

Usability testing is the systematic evaluation of the "interaction between people and the products, equipment, environments, and services they use" and "is the fundamental principle that underpins all ergonomics" (McClelland, 1990, p. 218). Usability testing also has been called user acceptance testing, user trials, or usability engineering. It is usually conducted by human factors engineers. The focus of usability testing is the user. Many products are developed by designers or engineers who assume their products are functional, easy to use, and acceptable. Often the basis for this assumption is the designer's knowledge or the fact that the designers can easily use the products themselves. Usability testing makes no such assumptions; it makes consumers the most important element in product design.

Usability testing typically focuses on evaluating the human-to-machine interface in product design. Examples include evaluating controls and displays on automobile consoles or in aircraft cockpits, designing user-friendly software, or designing human-to-computer interfaces. Usability testing also can be applied to products that are not considered machines, as in workstation design (Davies & Phillips, 1986; Stubler & Bernard, 1986). Both complex (anesthesia monitors and mammography machines) and simple (walkers and splints) medical and rehabilitation equipment can benefit from experimental evaluation that concentrates on the users. User testing may or may not be conducted by the equipment manufacturer. If such testing is not done, evaluation by a medical and human factors team or by medical and rehabilitation personnel can be beneficial. This testing ensures that such devices will be usable in the appropriate operational environment by the targeted user groups.

The Process

The first step in the usability testing process is to identify subject-matter experts (SMEs) and the user population (Figure 6–1, step 1). A SME is any person who is considered to be a valid judge, by virtue of his or her experience, education, or research, of system operations, job performance, or task dimensions. After the experts and users are identified, the investigators, SMEs, and representatives from the user group meet. During this meeting, the project is defined and questions about the product are raised through discussion (Figure 6–1, step 2). During this meeting, the groundwork is laid for development of design objectives and task and function analysis.

The next two steps, which can occur simultaneously, are to identify design objectives and to conduct a task and function analysis (Figure 6–1, steps 3 and 4). Design objectives focus on product features that affect performance, safety, expense, acceptance, comfort, ease of use, and aesthetics. Inclusion of these objectives in initial product development helps verify that the product is effective, safe, and accepted by user groups before an investment is made in expensive product construction. Once a product is in the manufacturing process, changes are not easy to implement. The design objectives should be closely related to the task and function analysis, and both are accomplished as a team effort among investigators, users, and SMEs.

The task and function analysis is used to develop the evaluation process. During a task and function analysis, the task to be performed is analyzed according to the aspects that are most demanding, frequent, and essential for accomplishing the goals. The analysis also identifies the pattern and sequence of tasks and subtasks.

The design objectives and the information from the task and function analysis are used for the fifth step, the development of performance criteria. Performance criteria should closely resemble the requirements of the task and should be performance-oriented (action-oriented). For example, a task analysis of an assembly job might indicate that fine-motor coordination is an important performance criterion.

Measurement techniques are chosen to quantify performance (Figure 6–1, step 6). These techniques include both objective and subjective measurements. Typical objective measurements include reaction time, number of errors, and type of error. Subjective measurements include user ratings of comfort, convenience, ease of use, and aesthetics.

Once the measurement techniques are chosen, subjects are recruited and trained (Figure 6–1, step 7). It is important to complete steps 1 through 6 before recruiting subjects to guarantee full disclosure of the evaluation process. It is recommended that a walk-through or trial of the evaluation process be conducted at this time.

Finally, the evaluation process is conducted as either a formal or an informal research project (Figure 6–1, step 8). The results are used to critique or redesign the product (Figure 6–1, step 9).

The process is iterative as new information becomes available or the design is changed. A design is proposed, tested, rejected (or accepted), and revised repeatedly (Meister, 1985). During the initial design and development, a number of prototypes may be developed and tested. Designs can be assessed through the use of paper-based product description, mock-ups,

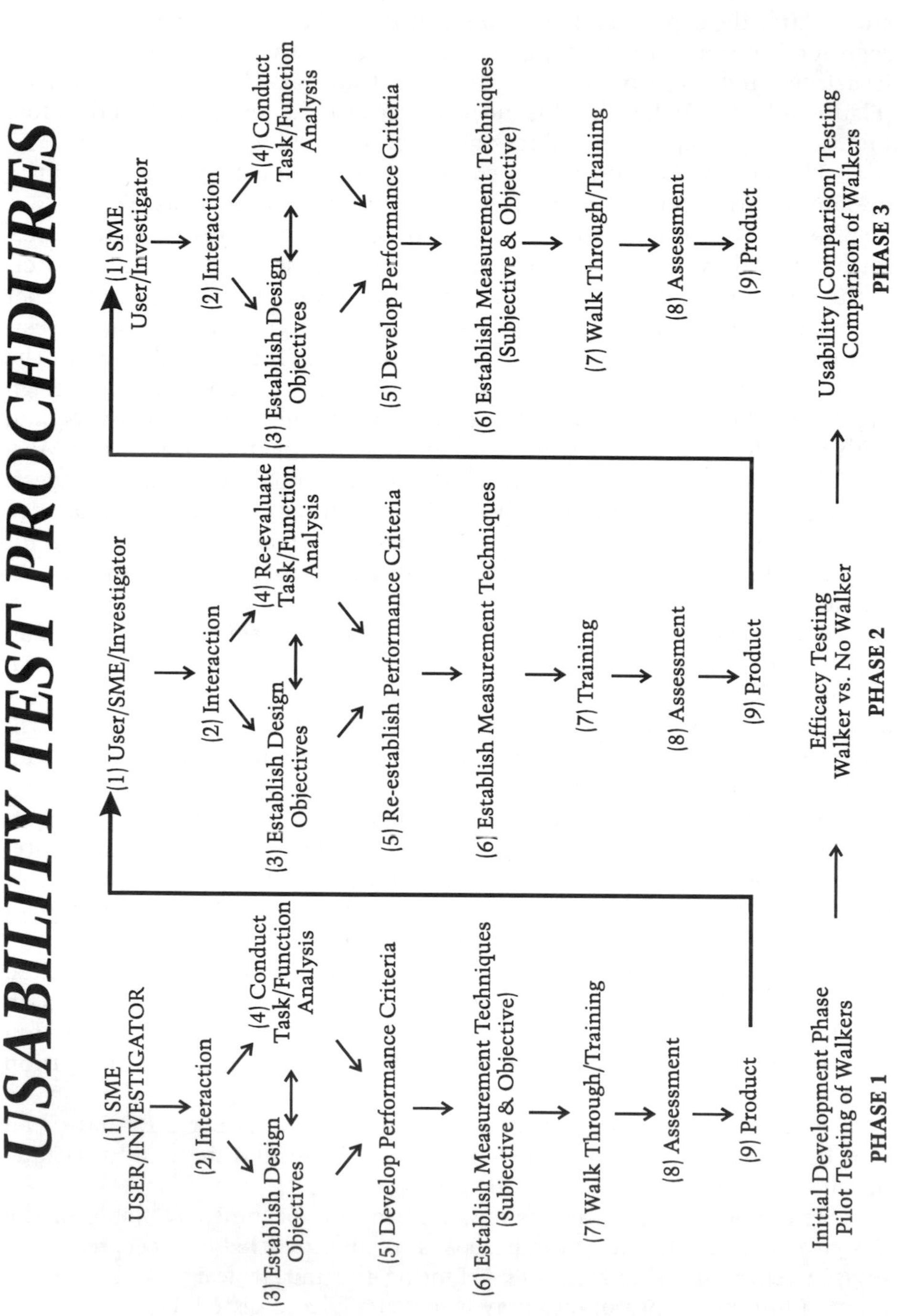

USABILITY TEST PROCEDURES

FIGURE 6–1 Usability test procedures. (SME stands for subject matter expert.)

prototypes (partial or full), or complete functional products. One or two design options are then chosen for rigorous evaluation. The evaluations can be categorized as experimental or nonexperimental, formal or informal, two-dimensional or three-dimensional, and nonperformance- or performance-oriented (Meister, 1985).

An experimental evaluation requires measurement of subject performance under contrasting conditions in a controlled environment and use of experimental and statistical controls. A nonexperimental evaluation does not require contrasting conditions or strict controls. For example, evaluating a subject's reaction time and subjective reaction to several versions of a product in a laboratory setting is experimental. Having subjects complete a subjective rating scale while using a product on the job is nonexperimental. Formal assessments have definite procedures and are well defined; informal assessments have less defined objectives and procedures. For example, a questionnaire is formal, but an open-ended group discussion is informal. Two-dimensional evaluations are static and are used to examine a product in terms of its attributes (checklists), whereas a three-dimensional evaluation may use mock-ups or prototypes and can incorporate either nonperformance or performance measurements (Meister, 1985).

An experimental evaluation of two or more prototype designs asks which design is better according to user performance and preference. If only one product is evaluated, the assessment addresses the same design questions of effectiveness, ease of use, accomplishment of the mission, and deficits or areas that need improvement, but only for that one product.

One important aspect of usability testing is that it is performed during each stage of development. However, even after the product is on the market, usability assessment can be conducted to ensure the product remains useful and effective. If product development occurred without usability testing, evaluation may be the first step in determining if change is needed. The user population, especially patients, may not believe they have the right, the knowledge, or the energy to voice their concerns about the effectiveness of a product. This leaves the responsibility with the developers and knowledgeable members of the medical user population (medical professionals who use, prescribe, or recommend products). The information gained from a usability evaluation after the product is on the market can determine the need for product redesign and assist medical personnel in making recommendations. Information regarding the effectiveness, efficiency, and ease of use of a product is important in the recommendation of a product for purchase by a client, a client's family, or a medical facility.

Product Development, Efficacy Testing, and Comparison Testing of a Client Walker

Many clients use walkers to increase mobility. Many types of walkers are available. Some have features such as baskets and pouches for carrying small items and drink holders. Some are balanced at the center handle; these walkers are designed for clients with hemiplegia and thus with limited use of one hand. Wheeled walkers may be especially beneficial during the early rehabilitation process, but it is difficult to know whether one with front wheels only or one with three wheels will best serve a client. Other important features are the weight, portability, and stability of the walker and the height, shape, and size of the grip handles.

For this example, a therapist (hereafter referred to as the investigator) has an idea for a new walker design. Three iterations of the usability process are needed. During the first iteration (product development) several variations of the new walker design are constructed and evaluated. This is prototype or pilot testing: both the walker design and the testing process are evaluated. The information gained from the pilot test is then used in the second iteration of the usability process, in which the best walker design (as determined during the pilot test) is evaluated (efficacy testing). This phase involves a more formal process of performance testing in a controlled setting to determine the effectiveness of the new walker. The final phase (comparison, or field, testing) consists of a field study to determine user acceptance and performance. This testing is conducted in a setting similar to the environment in which the walker will be used.

Although three titles are used for the three different phases, each phase is considered usability testing. Usability testing simply means that the product is evaluated by obtaining information from representative users while they use the product. The goals of usability testing are to develop a product that (1) fully accomplishes the purpose for which it was designed; (2) is easy to use; and (3) will be used. The third goal entails factors, such as aesthetics, that influence whether or not a person chooses to use the product. In addition, the best design is one that does not require the user to study an instruction manual. That is, the design should be intuitive and make sense to the user.

First Iteration: Product Development

The goal of product development is to produce several design alternatives and to select one for additional evaluation. The first step is to identify the SMEs, users, and investigators (Figure 6-1). This group could include product developers; medical personnel who have prescribed walkers for their clients; therapists and nurses who work closely with clients who use walkers; family members of clients who use walkers; and the clients themselves. A target group of clients should be identified, because the needs of various groups, such as clients with hemiplegia and clients with cerebral palsy, differ. For example, a client who has problems with balance and coordination may not want wheels on his or her walker, and a client who quickly becomes fatigued may need an attachable seat that folds while the patient is walking. For this example, a geriatric population is chosen.

The second step is the interactive process between the investigators and the SMEs and users (Figure 6–1). During this interaction, deficiencies in existing walker designs are identified and consequent research questions are developed. Positive aspects of existing walker designs may be identified and incorporated into the design objectives (Figure 6–1, step 3).

Design objectives are developed as a result of the observations, replies to questionnaires, and discussions among SMEs, users, and investigators (Table 6–1). Design objectives should include any items considered important to enable full, practical use of the walker. The development of design objectives should answer the question, "What design features are important for a walker to be used by this target population?" The purpose of a walker is to assist people in walking and allow them to stabilize themselves by putting some of their weight on the walker handles. Therefore, the first objective should be stability. Secondary characteristics of the design are those that are important to a user but that may not influence the primary purpose of the product. An example is making the walker easily collapsible for placing into a car. Tertiary items include attractiveness and convenience. Convenience characteristics of a walker might include baskets or pouches for personal items and attachable trays to hold food or drinks.

Labeling design objectives as primary, secondary, and tertiary does not mean one level is more important than another. Secondary and tertiary items are important because they influence whether or not the product will be accepted and used. A product may help clients accomplish a task but be so difficult, inconvenient, or unattractive to use that people choose to do without it. The importance of individual design objectives should be determined by the combined interaction of the SMEs, users, and investigators.

While design objectives are being defined, a task and function analysis should be accomplished (Figure 6–1, step 4). Information gained from establishing the design objectives should be used in conducting the task and function analysis and vice versa. The task and function analysis is based on input from users and SMEs. The investigator who conducts the assessment should observe the user performing a typical task and break the task into its component parts. These components should be described using action phrases. The design objectives and the information gained from the task and function analysis are used to develop performance criteria (Figure 6–1, step 5).

Representative tasks are identified on the basis of criticality, frequency, and difficulty. The selected tasks can be used as independent variables (the different walkers are also independent variables). For this situation, the tasks chosen could include (1) walking and maneuvering around items that block the user's path; (2) entering, using, and exiting a restroom; and (3) using a

Table 6–1 Design objectives for Product Development.

Primary Objectives:

Walker:
> Light weight
> Adjustable height
> Adjustable width
> Stability

Client:
> Appropriate weight distribution
> Ability to maintain erect posture during use

Secondary Objectives:

> Comfort
> Ease of use
> Ease of adjustment
> Ease of storage
> Portability
> Optimum grip height,
>   shape,
>   size

Tertiary Objectives:

> Attractiveness
> Convenience

---

small set of stairs. For this example, the first task is used to test the walker prototypes. Performance criteria are developed from the selected task.

The fifth step is to establish subjective and objective measurements. Because the first iteration is the development phase, it may be determined that only one task will be used to select the new design for the walker. In a similar manner, only the design objectives deemed most important may be used. The breadth and depth of the evaluation during the product-development stage are determined by the investigator. Consideration of costs and benefits assists the investigator in making the determination. For example, if construction of the walkers for additional testing is expected to be expensive, the testing should be thorough. If construction and possible alterations are relatively inexpensive, the prototype study may be smaller in terms of breadth and depth (or complexity).

Primary design objectives (dependent measurements) require both objective and subjective measurements. Dependent measurements for the sample situation are listed in Table 6–2. In addition to the measurements listed, the base and depth of the walker should be measured to determine walker stability. Many manufacturers list the weight capacity of walkers.

Table 6–2   Dependent Measurements for Product Development.

Objective

    Walker weight
    Height adjustment
    Percentage of the target population who can use the walker
    Distance between walker legs
    Biomechanical analysis of weight distribution
    Material strength

Subjective

    Perceived stability
    Perceived comfort
    Perceived pain or strain
    Perceived exertion
    Perceived ease of use
    Perceived ease of adjustment
    Perceived portability
    Forced-choice rankings

However, if more information is required, material strength can be determined through consultation with an engineer familiar with the materials and construction of walkers. Subjective measurement techniques may include interviews, questionnaires, rankings, Likert scale ratings, or ratings by means of techniques such as magnitude estimation (Cordes, 1984). Group interviews, rather than open-ended individual interviews, are often used to promote discussion and "co-discovery" (McClelland, 1990). Forced-choice rankings are especially useful in the comparison of several designs. Forced-choice rankings require the user to rank the designs in order of preference. Observations and ratings by the investigator can be helpful, but the investigator must take care not to bias the results.

Subject training and a walk-through of the testing process comprise the seventh step (Figure 6–1). Enough training should be done to eliminate a learning (or practice) effect. That is, subjects should not continue to improve with time, regardless of experimental condition.

The eighth step is the comparison study of several prototype walkers. Subjects perform one or more of the reference tasks, and the investigator collects and analyzes objective and subjective information. On the basis of the analysis, one design is usually selected for the next phase—efficacy testing. In the example, the walking task is evaluated in a nonexperimental, formal-informal, three-dimensional, and performance-oriented context. In this case, nonexperimental means no statistical controls, even though contrasting conditions are used (one walker design compared with another). The comparison study contains both formal and informal elements, because a formal procedure and questionnaire are used in addition to an informal interview session. The process is three-dimensional because prototypes of the walkers are used in a realistic task.

The goal of the evaluation (to identify one walker for additional testing) can be met with a relatively small number of participants. Subjects receive a detailed briefing, undergo a medical screening, and sign an informed consent form. Each hospital or nursing facility usually has a human-use committee that determines the requirements for briefing, screening, and the format and contents of the consent form.

In the example, the experimental design is a repeated-measurements design, counterbalanced for order. A repeated-measurements design means that each subject served as his or her own control and completed the task under each of the experimental conditions (various walker designs). Counterbalancing for the order in which each walker is used can be accomplished by using a balanced Latin-square design. This means each treatment condition (each walker design) is immediately preceded and followed once by each of the other conditions (Winer et al, 1991). This is often the preferred method to counterbalance a design without having to conduct tests of all possible ordering combinations. Another method of controlling for order effects is to randomize the order of administration using a random-number table.

Analysis of the subjective data can be accomplished by the use of nonparametric statistical analysis (Siegel, 1956; Winer et al, 1991). Nonparametric statistical analysis is a useful tool for usability studies that collect subjective data and employ small sample sizes. Parametric statistical analysis can be used for objective data when proper experimental design and sufficient population sampling are used to allow inference to the whole population. There is considerable debate over using parametric statistics with subjective data (Anderson, 1961; Gaito, 1987; Westermann, 1983).

The results should clearly indicate the preferred design on the basis of user preference and performance data. The investigator may give a weighting factor to items considered to be of primary importance. For example, object load (lbs.), adjustability, use by the greatest percentage of the target population, and biomechanical advantage may be given heavier weights than convenience and aesthetics.

As a result of the first iteration, design 1 is selected for additional testing (Table 6–3). This design is selected because it has the largest height range and is considered the most stable, adjustable, and portable. Its use caused the least pain and strain, and it was ranked the preferred walker.

Second Iteration: Efficacy Testing, Controlled Setting

The goal of efficacy testing is to determine whether the walker improves the user's ability to walk and maneuver through the activities of daily living. Therefore, testing consists of having subjects use the walker, as opposed to not using a walker, while performing several representative tasks. If the investigator believes that walkers have been shown to be effective ambula-

Table 6–3. Hypothetical Results from Product Development.

	Design 1	Design 2	Design 3
Load	6 lbs	7 lbs	16 lbs
Height	27" to 37"	32" to 37"	30" to 38"
Weight distribution	good	good	good
Material construction	350 lb capacity	375 lb capacity	500 lb capacity
Posture	good	good	good
Stability	17.5*	12.2	14.0
Comfort	14.5	15.8	16.0
Pain/Strain/ Discomfort	12.1*	14.2	14.6
Ease of Use	10.3	12.2	16.8*
Adjustment	18.7*	16.0	14.8
Portability	16.5*	13.9	9.8
Ranking	1.25*	2.25	2.50

*Significantly different from other two walkers (p < 0.05) All ratings (except ranking) used a Borg-type scale with anchored subjective ratings 0-20 (Borg, 1962). The lower number indicates less and the higher number indicates more of the given quality. Rankings were 1-3.

tion tools in the past and that such an evaluation would be superfluous, this phase can be eliminated. If this phase is eliminated, usability testing begins with a comparison between the new design and existing designs (usability [comparison] testing, Figure 6–1, Phase 3).

Identification of the SMEs and users was accomplished in the beginning of phase 1 (pilot testing); the experimental subjects now are added to the group as SMEs (Figure 6–1, step 1). The interaction among SMEs, users, and the investigator should focus on the results of the pilot test (Figure 6–1, step 2).

The design objectives for the walker most likely will remain the same as those identified in the development phase (Table 6–1; Figure 6–1, step 3). However, additional objectives can be identified in the pilot testing and in the interactions among the subjects, SMEs, and users.

The task and function analysis should be reevaluated (Figure 6–1, Phase 2, step 4). The representative tasks can be altered on the basis of information gained during the development phase. For the second iteration of the process—efficacy testing—all three representative tasks are used to ascertain whether or not the new walker meets the functional goals. The tasks identified during the task or functional analysis are (1) walking and maneuvering around items that block the user's path; (2) entering, using, and exiting a restroom, and (3) using a small set of stairs. In each task, performance criteria should be measurable. They should provide information essential to successful performance and should include objective and subjective data (Figure 6–1, step 5). When the same criteria are used for product development,

Table 6–4. Hypothetical Results from Efficacy Testing: Walking and Maneuvering Task.

	Walker	*No Walker*
Total Time	9.2 min	15.6 min
get up	1.0 min	2 min
turn right	.45 min	1.2 min
walk 5 ft	1.5 min	2.6 min
walk around chair	.60 min	1.5 min
walk 4 ft	1.3 min	2.0 min
avoid toy	1 min	1.9 min
walk 5 ft	1.77 min	2.9 min
sit in chair	1.4 min	1.5 min
Heart Rate	145 beats/min	155 beats/min
Perceived Exertion	15.8*	18.3
Stability	19.7*	5.1
Comfort	18.5*	6.7
Pain/Strain	5.5*	14.2

*Significantly different from no walker ($p < 0.05$). All ratings (except ranking) used a Borg-type scale with anchored subjective ratings 0 to 20 (Borg, 1962). The lower number indicates less and the higher number indicates more of the given quality.

efficacy testing, and comparison testing, performance standards can be developed and product improvement can be monitored over time. Additional dependent measurements in the example include time to complete each element of the task, time to complete the entire procedure, heart rate, and perceived exertion (Borg, 1962; 1970; 1978, Table 6–4).

In the example, the same objective and subjective measurement techniques used during the development phase are used during efficacy testing (Table 6–2; Figure 6–1, step 6). The first task is walking and maneuvering around items that block the user's path. This task involves the following procedures: rising from an easy chair; turning right; walking 5 feet and maneuvering to the left of a chair that blocks the path; walking 4 feet and maneuvering right to avoid a child's toy; walking another 5 feet; and sitting in a kitchen chair.

In addition to the primary task of walking, important secondary tasks should be included in the testing procedure. For example, if the walker is used to enable someone to move between a desk and a filing cabinet, such a task pattern should be incorporated into the testing procedure.

Again, subjects should be trained in each task used in the test procedure (Figure 6–1, step 7). Because more than one procedural task (walking, maneuvering in a restroom, and using stairs) is being studied, the order of the tasks should be balanced to control for order effects, such as transfer of learning or a conditioning effect. Training of test subjects in testing procedures also decreases the likelihood that learning effects will occur and influence the study results.

After training, the actual assessment (experimental evaluation) takes place. Task performance should be evaluated by means of timing and accuracy data. In the example, efficacy testing is experimental, formal, three-dimensional performance testing. As with any research method, consistency in experimental testing must be ensured in subject training, measurement techniques, and data compilation. Two excellent resources on these topics are Winer et al (1991) for laboratory studies and Cook and Campbell (1979) for field studies.

During efficacy testing, the number of subjects will probably be greater than the number who participated in the pilot test. Adequate results can be obtained with a relatively small number of subjects, especially because this is a repeated-measurements study. Statistical analysis can include a repeated-measurements analysis of variance (ANOVA) and post hoc testing.

The results should give the investigator clear information about the efficacy of use of the walker, as opposed to no walker, in terms of both the subjects' performance and their preference. Efficacy testing provides information on the benefits and limitations of using the walker in three different situations for men and women. Hypothetical results reveal that the walker is beneficial (Table 6–4). The subjects performed the task more quickly, experienced less subjective exertion, less pain and strain, more stability, more comfort, and had a lower heart rate when they used the walker than when they did not use the walker. The final output is the product (Figure 6–1, step 9), which is reevaluated by the research team.

Third Iteration: Comparison Field Testing

The second iteration of the usability cycle (efficacy testing) revealed that the walker was helpful in improving ambulation and maneuvering and in using a restroom. However, the following concerns were identified during testing:

1. The gripping edge of the walker was uncomfortable and caused pain on the thenar eminence during ambulation.
2. Subjects requested a handle material that does not feel cold to touch and comes in different colors.
3. Subjects requested detachable accessories, such as a tray for holding objects, a recessed cup holder, and a basket with adjustable sections.
4. The fold-up seat was weak and unstable and did not have appropriate contour or padding.

The concerns must be discussed by SMEs, subjects, users, and investigators (Figure 6–1, steps 1 and 2). The cost of product development and the purchase price must be considered along with the preferences expressed. The changes that can be made are incorporated into the design objectives, and a new walker is constructed (Figure 6–1, step 3). The new design must then be reevaluated in the type of environment in which it is to be used. In addition, the investigator should compare this design with that of other walkers available on the commercial market (usability [comparison] testing, Figure 6–1, Phase 3).

A review of the task and function analysis reveals that the assistance provided by the walker is most pronounced during the walking task. Because both the old and the new design objectives can be tested with the walking task, this task is chosen as the representative task (Figure 6–1, step 4). The purpose of the comparison field testing is to compare one or more designs with each other in a realistic environment. Should the investigator choose to do so, he or she can compare the findings obtained when a subject uses the new walker design with the findings obtained when no walker is used to verify the results of the efficacy test in a realistic environment.

The task in comparison testing should be similar to the task used during efficacy testing in the laboratory. The tests can be conducted in a nursing home where throw rugs, narrow halls, and wheel chairs serve as obstructions. It can also be conducted in a work setting where storage cabinets are located in the halls, ramps are located between split-level floors, and where there is low-level ambient light. The most appropriate setting for the target group is determined by the users, SMEs, and the investigator. Again, if users are required to perform additional tasks or carry objects, these tasks are included in the evaluation (Figure 6–1, step 5). The objective and subjective measurement techniques are the same as those used during efficacy testing in order to verify results (Figure 6–1, step 6).

Training and a walk-through of the test situation are conducted because the conditions have changed from a laboratory-based evaluation to a field test. Once again, training helps prevent mistakes during testing and serves to eliminate a learning effect (Figure 6–1, step 7). The assessment is the eighth step, and applying the data obtained to the product design is the ninth step.

The results of the comparison test in the example are as follows: The new design was ranked as the preferred walker compared with the other two walkers. The subjects' heart rates were lower with the new design. Subjects completed the task faster when they used the new design; however, time to stand and sit was slower. Subjects found the new design easier to use. Use of the new design increased comfort and decreased pain and strain. No differences were found for ratings of stability, perceived exertion, or performance of ancillary tasks. These results showed the new design to be superior for ambulatory assistance as measured by user preference and performance (Table 6–5).

Table 6–5 Hypothetical Results of Walker Subjective Ratings.

	New Design	*Walker A*	*Walker B*
Stability	18.8	17.7	19.0
Comfort	15.3*	12.3	14.0
Pain/Strain	8.9*	17.3	16.2
Ease of Use	15.0	15.9	16.5
Perceived Exertion	16.4	15.0	15.2
Ranking	1.25*	2.5	2.25

*Significantly different from other two walkers (p < 0.05). All ratings (except ranking) used a Borg-type scale with anchored subjective ratings 0-20 (Borg, 1962). A lower number indicates less and a higher number indicates more of the indicated quality. Rankings are 1-3.

Conclusion

Usability testing of medical or rehabilitation equipment is an essential component of product development, but it is often neglected. This neglect becomes obvious when practitioners or clients attempt to use the product. Without user testing, products are often difficult to use, cannot be used intuitively, are not comfortable, and are not made for all users, such as technicians, medical practitioners, and clients. The importance of usability testing of medical equipment has become widely recognized, as evidenced by its consideration as one criterion for approving products and setting international and national standards (McClelland, 1990). One example cited by McClelland (1990) is the British standard for reclosable pharmaceutical containers.

Medical professionals often design equipment on the basis of their experience with clients or according to individual client needs, but they fail to complete the design sequence by conducting systematic user tests. Rather than having factual knowledge of the success of the product, they have two sets of opinions (their own and those of the clients with whom they work). As such, there is little ability to generalize the effectiveness to a broad client population.

Usability testing provides a mechanism to evaluate a product from a user's perspective. The procedure should be used to assess all rehabilitation and medical equipment. Manufacturers, practitioners, and instructors in professional programs should begin introducing the concepts and procedures of usability testing to improve client care.

References

Anderson, N.H. (1961). Scales and statistics: Parametric and nonparametric. Psychological Bulletin, 58:305-316.

Borg, G.A. (1962). Physical Performance and Perceived Exertion. Lund, Sweden: Gleerup.

Borg, G.A. (1970). Perceived exertion as an indicator of somatic stress. Scandinavian Journal of Rehabilitation Medicine, 2:92-98.

Borg, G.A. (1978). Subjective aspects of physical and mental load. Ergonomics, 21:215-220.

Cook, T.T., Campbell, D.T. (1979). Quasi-experimentation: Design and Analysis Issues for Field Settings. Boston: Houghton Mifflin.

Cordes, R.E. (1984). Use of magnitude estimation for evaluating product ease-of-use. In E. Grandjean (Ed.), Ergonomics and Health in Modern Offices. New York: Taylor & Francis.

Davies, D.K., and Phillips, M.D. (1986). Assessing user acceptance of next generation air traffic controller workstations. In Proceedings of the Human Factors Society, 30th Annual Meeting, Sept. 29-October 3, Dayton, Ohio. Santa Monica: Human Factors Society.

Gaito, J. (1987). Measurement scales and statistics: Resurgence of an old misconception. Psychological Bulletin, 101:159-165.

McClelland, I. (1990). Product assessment and user trials. In J.R. Wilson & E.N. Corlett (Eds.), Evaluation of Human Work: A Practical Ergonomics Methodology. New York: Taylor & Francis.

Meister, D. (1985). Behavioral Analysis and Measurement Methods. New York: Wiley.

Meister, D. (1989). Conceptual Aspects of Human Factors. Baltimore: Johns Hopkins University Press.

Siegel, S. (1956). Nonparametric Statistics for the Behavioral Sciences. New York: McGraw-Hill.

Stubler, W.F., Bernard, T.E. (1986). Office ergonomics: Design methodology and evaluation. In Proceedings of the Human Factors Society, 30th Annual Meeting, Sept. 29- Oct. 3, Dayton, Ohio. Santa Monica: Human Factors Society.

Westermann, R. (1983). Interval-scale measurement of attitudes: Some theoretical conditions and empirical testing methods. British Journal of Mathematics and Statistical Psychology, 36:228-239.

Winer, B.J., Brown, D.R., Michels, K.M. (1991). Statistical Principles in Experimental Design. New York: McGraw-Hill.

Suggested Reading

Bailey, R.W. (1982). Human Performance Engineering. Englewood Cliffs, N.J.: Prentice Hall.

Benel, D.C.R., Pain, R.F. (1985). The human factors usability laboratory in product evaluation. In Proceedings of the Human Factors Society, 29th Annual Meeting, October, Baltimore, Md. Santa Monica: Human Factors Society.

Brown, C.R., Schaum, D.L. (1980). User-adjusted VDU parameters. In E. Grandjean & E. Vigliani (Eds.), Ergonomic Aspects of Visual Display Terminals. New York: Taylor & Francis.

Kantowitz, B.H., Sorkin, R.D. (1983). Human Factors: Understanding People-system Relationships. New York: Wiley.

Salvendy, G. (Ed.) (1987). Handbook of Human Factors. New York: Wiley.

Shneiderman, B. (1987). Designing the User Interface: Strategies for Effective Human-computer Interaction. Reading, Mass.: Addison-Wesley.

Whiteside, J., Bennett, J., Holtzblatt, K. (1988). Usability Engineering: Our Experience and Evolution. In M. Helander (Ed.), Handbook of Human-Computer Interaction. Amsterdam: North Holland.

PART III

Special Considerations

CHAPTER 7

Lifting Testing and Analysis

Joann Brooks

ABSTRACT

The task of lifting is one of the most common physical demands in industrial settings. Industrial injuries related to lifting are the second most common reason cited for back injury after slips and falls. The variables of lifting can be categorized into physical, environmental, and psychologic. The physical variables of the object lifted include size, weight, distribution of weight, horizontal and vertical distance lifted, and handles. Environmental variables include the time of day, frequency and duration of lifting, temperature, lighting, clothing, and friction coefficients of working surfaces. Psychologic variables include perceived effort, stress, safety awareness, and work attitudes. All variables are important in determining lifting ability. Lifting ability can be tested by isokinetic, isometric, isoinertial, and psychophysical methods. All methods have advantages and disadvantages. A dynamic lifting test is a model for determining lifting ability in the workplace.

Despite extensive research, testing, training, and education, close to 400,000 new cases of work-related disabling injuries and disease occur each year in the United States (Elling, 1989). Injuries to the lower part of the back are the leading musculoskeletal disorder. In 1987 these injuries accounted for more than 85% of all claims for worker compensation, according to the National Safety Council (Elling, 1989). Overexertion is the leading cause of injury in industry today, and 68% of overexertion incidents involve lifting (Liles & Mahajan, 1985).

Lifting methods and factors have been studied extensively. Numerous contributions and recommendations have been made to industry and to rehabilitation specialists to minimize the risk of injury or reinjury to people who lift at work. Many lifting standards and guidelines have been developed to promote safe habits in the workplace and at home. Testing methods have been developed to aid in determining a worker's ability or readiness to perform lifting tasks. Unfortunately, most lifting-ability tests are limited to measuring one of two factors that affect lifting performance. The inability to capture the complex interactions of all the factors that affect lifting result in poor to fair prediction of work ability or potential for injury.

This chapter provides an overview of the many factors to be considered in the evaluation and design of and training for lifting tasks in an attempt to provide safe working conditions for both uninjured and injured workers. The advantages and disadvantages of lifting methods and analyses are compared. The therapist should be able to choose suitable methods for testing and training on the basis of the individual needs of the worker.

Lifting Injuries

Lifting injuries can be classified into three groups: accidental, due to overexertion, and cumulative (Pheasant, 1991).

Accidental injuries occur when a load is heavier or lighter than expected; contents of the load shift during lifting; the coupling between the hands and the load is released; footing is lost or the worker slips on the work surface; and or interference occurs during the lift. This type of injury is difficult to prevent with traditional training and education. These injuries account for one-third of all injuries despite administrative and engineering controls (Liles & Mahajan, 1985; Snook & White, 1984). Constant monitoring and quality improvements are the best way to prevent injuries of this nature.

Injuries due to overexertion are considered the most frequent of all work-related injuries (National Institute for Occupational Safety and Health [NIOSH], 1981; Pheasant, 1991; Sapega, 1990). These injuries cause muscular strain, ligamentous sprains, annular tears in the intervertebral disk, joint sprains, and other soft-tissue injuries when the physical properties of the tissues are exceeded by excessive forces, durations, or combinations of both. Most injuries due to overexertion can be prevented with safe and biomechanically sound approaches to lifting at work, which are matched with the physical characteristics of the worker (Sapega, 1990).

Cumulative injuries are the most complicated of all lifting injuries to prevent and manage. The cumulative effect of subclinical injuries to the joint cartilage, ligaments, disks, and muscles is usually detected at a late stage (Noone & Mazumdar, 1992). Degenerative disk disease and osteoarthrosis are common findings in the medical evaluation of acute lifting injuries (NIOSH, 1981). The relation between contributing factors of heredity, work demands, aging, trauma, and other physical demands is not well understood. Although poor work habits over the years are considered contributory to many lifting injuries, a young worker who has no symptoms is difficult to retrain. Cumulative trauma is currently an area of interest to industry and the focus of many industrial injury-prevention programs (Elling, 1989).

Factors That Affect Lifting Ability

Sex

In general, men are considered to be stronger than women. The strength of the average woman is considered to be approximately 60% of the strength of the average man. Caution must be used in this generalization because of the wide range of strengths among both men and women (NIOSH, 1981). Differences in spinal compression tolerance are a result of the smaller force-bearing areas of the vertebral bodies of women (Bejjani et al, 1984). The type of forces generated at the spine during lifting differ between men and women. Shear forces are more characteristic of the spine of women because women have higher lumbosacral angles than men; compression forces are more characteristic of the spine of men (Bejjani et al, 1984).

Body Weight

Body weight must be considered in lifting. The head, neck, trunk, and arms account for approximately 68.8% of the total body weight (Dempster, 1955). Once an object is lifted, the weight of the head, neck, trunk, and arms must be added to the weight of the object to determine the total force and lifting moment. Body weight is not a good predictor of lifting strength because there are large variations in the relative quantities of fat and lean body mass (Batti'e et al, 1989a). A high body weight can be an advantage in lifting heavier loads, in which a large mass can counterbalance a large load. However, a high body weight can be a disadvantage in repetitive lifting. A high body weight increases the metabolic rate and can cause early fatigue unless the worker has undergone endurance training (NIOSH, 1981).

Table 7–1. Classification of Strength Requirements for Lifting.

Type of Work	Load (lb [kg])		Frequency of Lifting
Sedentary	≤ 10	(4.5)	Infrequent
Light	≤ 20	(9.0)	Infrequent
	≤ 10	(4.5)	Frequent
Medium	≤ 50	(22.7)	Infrequent
	≤ 25	(11.4)	Frequent
Heavy	≤ 100	(45.4)	Infrequent
	≤ 50	(22.7)	Frequent
Very Heavy	> 100	(45.4).	Infrequent
	> 50	(22.7).	Frequent

Age

Age has been negatively correlated with both strength and the incidence of work-related injuries (Batti'e et al, 1989b). In general, strength declines after 40 years of age. At the age of 65 years, strength is 75 to 85% of the maximum value. The rate and extent of the decline of strength with age are related to the amount of exercise and type of lifestyle (Pheasant, 1991). With the aging of the work force, greater consideration needs to be given to the strength and tolerances of aging tissues to withstand physically demanding workloads.

Factors That Affect Lifting

Weight of the Object

The importance of the weight of the object depends on the size of the object, the location of the object, the vertical and horizontal distances the object is moved, and the frequency of lifting. The United States Department of Labor classifies strength requirements for tasks on the basis of the weight of the object and in the general categories of frequent and infrequent lifting (Matheson & Ogden, 1983). Maximum values of weight are given for frequent and infrequent lifting within each category (Table 7–1).

When a task is classified, the higher category is always chosen. Caution should be used when one bases the level of work capacity on the weight of the object. Factors such as the size of the object and the location, frequency, and duration of lifting can affect the classification of level of work.

Horizontal Distance

NIOSH considers horizontal distance a critical factor in determining the recommended weight limit for lifting. The greater the horizontal distance, the greater are the frequency and severity of musculoskeletal injuries (An-

dersson et al, 1976; Chaffin & Park, 1973). The horizontal distance is measured from the center of the object to the center of the ankles (NIOSH, 1981).
The horizontal distance also corresponds to the moment arm between the
center of the object and the center of the spine. NIOSH recommends a
horizontal distance of 25 cm, which reflects the minimum distance in lifting
that will not interfere with the front of the body. The maximum horizontal
distance should not exceed 30 cm, which is beyond the reach of most people
(Putz-Anderson & Waters, 1991).

Size of the Object

The size of the object contributes to the horizontal distance and to the
moment arm during lifting (NIOSH, 1981). The larger the object, the larger
are the moment arm and the resulting forces generated during lifting. If an
object is too large to fit between the legs, the trunk must bend to reduce the
horizontal distance to minimize the lifting forces at the spine (Drury et al,
1982; Pheasant, 1991).

Vertical Location

The vertical location is determined by the location of the hands at the
beginning of the lift measured from the floor (NIOSH, 1981). The ideal
vertical location is between knuckle height and waist height (Pheasant,
1991). NIOSH recommends a maximum value for vertical location of 75 cm,
which corresponds to the average reach height (NIOSH, 1981).

Vertical Distance

The location of the object at the beginning and end of the lift determines the
vertical distance. The ideal lift occurs between knuckle height and waist
height (NIOSH, 1981; Pheasant, 1991). The acceptable maximum weight
then decreases in accordance with the following vertical distances (Jiang &
Ayoub, 1987; Waikar et al, 1991):

Floor to Knuckle Height	Highest Acceptable Maximum Weight
Knuckle to Shoulder Height	
Floor to Shoulder Height	
Floor to Reach Height	
Shoulder to Reach Height	Lowest Acceptable MaximumWeight

Symmetry of Lift

The location of the object in relation to the orientation of the body determines
the symmetry of lifting. Lifting in the sagittal plane of the body is ideal. In a
survey on box handling, symmetric lifting in the sagittal plane was the

exception (Drury et al, 1982). Asymmetric lifting is associated with many musculoskeletal injuries. Asymmetric loading of the trunk muscles leads to strain as the trunk muscles try to stabilize and balance the load on the spine (Kumar, 1984). The twisting associated with asymmetric lifting results in compression and torsional stresses on the spine, causing injury primarily to the facet joints and the disks (Farfan, 1970). Asymmetric lifting is also perceived as more fatiguing than symmetric lifting, according to a study that looked at lifting in 30-degree and 60-degree angles of displacement from the sagittal plane (Kumar, 1984). If load and the lift are not in the same plane, the trunk and pelvis should always be oriented in the plane of the object by a change in foot placement. Pivoting the feet avoids twisting at the trunk and twisting at the knees.

Frequency and Duration of Lifting

NIOSH classifies frequency of lifting by considering the rate of lifting per minute and the duration of time spent lifting at a specific rate (NIOSH, 1981; Putz-Anderson & Waters, 1991). Infrequent lifting is defined as less than 0.2 lifts per minute. High-frequency lifting is defined as 0.2 or more lifts per minute. Short duration refers to continuous lifting for up to 1 hour, followed by a recovery period of at least 120% of work time. Moderate duration refers to continuous lifting for up to 2 hours, followed by a recovery period of at least 30% of work time. Long duration refers to fatigue allowances other than those normally given during a work shift (NIOSH, 1981; Putz-Anderson & Waters, 1991).

Frequent lifting is associated with more incidents of musculoskeletal injury than infrequent lifting. Frequent lifting increases exposure to physical stressors that can accelerate degenerative wear and tear on the tissues, lack of coordination, and muscle fatigue. Workers have been found to prefer working at a fast pace with light loads over working at a slow pace with heavy loads to achieve the same work (Nicholson & Legg, 1986).

The training and rehabilitation of workers who lift frequently differ from those of workers who lift only occasionally. All lifting requires adequate strength and flexibility. With repetitive lifting, the additional requirements of endurance training and pacing with adequate recovery time must be added to training. Previously injured workers with degenerative disk and joint disease may require additional recovery time and modification of the rate of lifting, depending on tissue tolerance for frequent lifting.

Coupling

Coupling is defined as the hand-to-object contact or gripping method. In industry, few boxes have handles, and even when handles are present, they seldom are used (Drury et al, 1982). The most common positioning of the hands used in lifting is with one hand on the upper front corner and the other hand on the lower rear corner of the object (Drury et al, 1982). This position appears to provide the best horizontal and vertical stabilization.

Factors of weight, horizontal distance, vertical location, vertical distance, symmetry, frequency, and coupling are considered in determining the recommended weight limits for lifting in the revised 1991 NIOSH guidelines for manual lifting. Each variable is entered into an equation to determine the recommended weight limit (RWL). If the actual weight exceeds the RWL, adjustments of the task variables are recommended to reduce the risk for a lifting injury for that task (Putz-Anderson & Waters, 1991).

The 1991 NIOSH guidelines revised the definition of the location of the object in lifting to include symmetry of lifting. The standard lifting location is defined as a three-dimensional reference point for evaluating lifting posture. It consists of a vertical height of 75 cm, a horizontal distance of 25 cm, and location in the sagittal plane (Putz-Anderson & Waters, 1991). The 1991 NIOSH guidelines also revised the value for the maximum weight value based on the revised higher value for the horizontal distance (see Chapter 8 for a more detailed discussion). The maximum weight value (load constant) for the standard lifting location given selected conditions and constraints for a single lift is 23 kg (51 pounds) (Putz-Anderson & Waters, 1991).

Biomechanical Factors in Lifting

Speed and Acceleration

All lifting should be performed at a controlled pace to reduce acceleration. Acceleration of the object occurs very early in the lift, 150-200 msec into the lift (Gagnon & Smyth, 1992). If an object is being lifted to chest level and above, another phase of acceleration occurs that corresponds to the change in hand placement (Pheasant, 1991). Acceleration increases the peak forces during a lift and can cause microfractures at the vertebral body endplates, even when light loads are lifted (Patterson et al, 1987). Acceleration occurs with both the lift of the object and the extension of the trunk. High values of stress on the lower part of the back due to fast acceleration of the trunk have been recorded; this finding did not necessarily correlate with how quickly the load was lifted (Patterson et al, 1987).

To minimize the acceleration effects on the lower part of the back in lifting, the object should initially be lifted with a concentric contraction by the muscles of the thigh. Once the object is lifted with the legs, the weight of the object and the upper body is momentarily balanced by an eccentric contraction of the trunk extensors. This eccentric contraction is followed by a concentric contraction of the trunk extensors as the load and body weight are lifted in a combination of knee and trunk extension. The purpose of this sequence is to control the extent and velocity of movement of the trunk to minimize the peak values for trunk movement and spinal forces during lifting (Patterson et al, 1987).

The concept of delaying trunk extension at the initial phase of lifting is observed consistently in experienced weight lifters regardless of the weight of the load (Patterson et al, 1987). Inexperienced lifters begin a lift immediately with a concentric contraction of the trunk, which results in dangerously high moments and compression forces in the lower part of the back even when light loads are lifted. Lifting training programs should emphasize recognition of the effects of acceleration with immediate trunk extension. Training regimens should include lifting loads of varying weights to practice a consistent lifting sequence with control of the object from pick-up to placement.

Joint Angles

The maximum joint angles necessary for lifting have been measured for the lumbar spine (60 degrees), hips (125 degrees), knees (140 degrees), and ankles (25 degrees) (Bejjani et al, 1984; Pheasant, 1991). The angles of the joints required for a specific lift vary with the vertical height, horizontal distance, vertical distance, and the weight of the object. Optimum joint angles at the lumbar spine and the knees are most important. Increased forces measured at the patellofemoral joint, tibiofemoral joint, and the lumbar spine with some lifting postures are attributed to the development of degenerative arthrosis and degenerative disk disease (Noone & Mazumdar, 1992). The anthropometric characteristics of the person and the physiologic status of the joints must be considered in the determination of the optimum lifting position.

Lifting Style

Various lifting styles have been studied and recommended to minimize stressors on the lower part of the back. Studies of the stressors on the patellofemoral, ankle, and shoulder joints have shown no one style of lifting that can minimize the stressors at all joints. Changes in joint angles and trunk inclination vary as a function of the location, size, and weight of the load (Bejjani et al, 1984; Gracovetsky et al, 1990; Kumar & Davis, 1983).

Back lift or stoop lift

A back or stoop lift is performed with the knees straight and the back flexed. This lifting style is the least energy-consuming and requires the least amount of lower-extremity strength (Troup, 1977). It is commonly used for lifting objects of light to moderate weight, especially in repetitive lifting of short duration, as in stocking shelves or stacking objects. Using this style is more likely to result in ligamentous strain due to hyperflexion (Adams & Hutton,

1982) or muscular sprain and disk injuries due to high acceleration forces with trunk extension (Troup, 1977).

Leg lift, crouch lift, or deep squat

A leg lift is performed with the knees bent greater than 90 degrees and the back in a lordotic posture (Blankenship & Blankenship, 1986; Hebert & Miller, 1987; Tichauer, 1971; Troup, 1977). The lifter stands with feet flat, on the balls of the feet, or a combination of these positions, depending on the flexibility of the soleus muscle and ankle joint. This style of lifting is the most energy-consuming and requires considerable strength of the quadriceps and gluteal muscles to lift the combined load and the torso (Kumar, 1984; Noe et al, 1990). It is commonly used for lifting low-lying loads and heavy loads. The base of support may be wide to straddle compact loads, or the load may be placed in front of the knees if it is too wide to fit between the legs. Using this style places considerable stress on the patellofemoral joints and can contribute to degenerative changes in the cartilage on the surfaces of the patella and femur (Bejjani et al, 1984). When the worker has a small base of support or poor foot placement, imbalance can occur.

Trunk kinetic lift

A trunk kinetic lift is performed in the deep squat position, but the hips and pelvis are raised before the load is lifted, usually because of inadequate quadriceps strength to extend the knees while lifting the body and the weight of the load (Troup, 1977).

Two-stage leg lift or leg roll

A two-stage leg lift is performed in the deep squat position or semi-kneeling position. The weight is transferred to one or both thighs, held close to the body, and then raised vertically with the body as in the leg lift. This style is used with low-lying heavy and bulky objects in which strength is inadequate or the back needs to be protected from stress. This is a safe technique to use with a previously injured back (Blankenship & Blankenship, 1986; Troup, 1977).

Freestyle or partial squat

A partial squat is performed with the knees between 0 degrees of extension and 90 degrees of flexion. The back is in lordosis. This method is the most commonly used. The position of the back and knees varies with the size, width, weight, and vertical location of the object. This is considered the strongest and least tiring lift (for nonprofessional weight lifters) because the lifter uses a combination of lower-extremity and trunk strength (Andersson et al, 1976; Kumar, 1984). Using this style can place stress on the lower part of the back and knees depending on the lifter's coordination and control of the object during the lift.

In ideal situations, the style chosen for any lift should minimize the horizontal distance, minimize the overall energy cost, and minimize stress to most of the joints of the body. Strength requirements of the quadriceps, hip extensor, trunk extensor, and abdominal muscles and mobility requirements of the trunk, hip, knee, and ankle vary with the different styles. In choosing the proper lifting method in training, the instructor should emphasize principles of body mechanics rather than lifting technique. The trainee should be able to apply the principles learned to any lifting situation. The important points to emphasize are as follows:

Slow control of the object throughout the lift

Symmetric lifting in the sagittal plane

No twisting of the trunk

Wide base of support with feet flat

Load close to the body throughout the lift

Physiologic and Pathophysiologic Consideration of the Spine

Although lifting injuries include the shoulder, knee, and other areas of the body, the spine is the structure most frequently injured (Kumar, 1984). The mechanism of injury to the spine during lifting is complex. Preexisting pathologic conditions and degenerative disk and joint disease often are present, and they alter healing and recovery from injury. Many structures can be injured with residual effects that can affect performance and produce potential for reinjury if not considered in the rehabilitation, retraining, and reentry to work.

Muscular Strain

Muscular strain of the erector spinae group is a common diagnosis related to lifting injuries due to overexertion. The multisegmental spinal muscles bear the greatest load of all lumbar muscles because of their potential to produce large moments at the spine during lifting (McGill & Norman, 1986; Pope, 1987). Tenderness and swelling in the thoracic, sacral, and iliac regions correspond to injuries to the musculotendinous and tendinous attachments of the erector spinae muscles. Once the muscle soreness resolves, rehabilitation should focus on muscle strengthening and endurance to avoid chronic strain.

Ligamentous Strain

Ligamentous strain to the supraspinous, interspinous, iliolumbar, and sacro-iliac ligaments occurs in relation to lifting injuries. Ligamentous strain is associated with hyperflexion injuries to the lumbar spine and torsional strains on the pelvis. The strain occurs as a result of unexpected loading or when the load is beyond a safe distance for normal and controlled muscle contraction (Pope, 1987). Ligament healing is a long process. Early mobilization with protected loading is important to promote healing and strengthening of the ligament (Pope, 1987).

Disk Injury

Disk injuries result from repeated compression, torsion, and tensile forces generated during lifting. Microfracturing of the vertebral endplate has been identified with high extensor moments of the erector spinae group. Fracturing of the endplates and subchondral bone or vertebral bodies alters the metabolism and fluid imbibition to the disk, which leads to degeneration and fibrosis of the annular fibers of the disk. Compression, torsion, and tensile stresses lead to distal radial and circumferential fissuring in the annular fibers. Progressive tearing leads to annular bulging and the risk of herniation, extrusion, and protrusion of nuclear material (Gordon et al, 1990; Hampton et al, 1989; NIOSH, 1981). Degenerated disks display a higher creep rate and greater deformation under load and reach a state of equilibrium sooner than do normal disks. Recovery from the creep effect is inversely related to the duration of loading; it can take up to 20 hours (Kazarian, 1975). Severely degenerated disks may not recover fully overnight. This may affect performance in work-hardening programs and the worker's ability to return to a productive work schedule.

Spondylosis

Spondylosis or spinal stenosis may result from chronic degenerative disk disease with compromise of the spinal cord or nerve roots. The effects of flexion and extension combined with loading need to be considered in the determination of posturing and lifting techniques (NIOSH, 1981).

Facet Arthrosis

Facet arthrosis occurs as a result of trauma to the joint cartilage and capsule from continuous compression or tensile forces. Direct trauma to the joint occurs when the specific range of motion is exceeded. Facet arthrosis also accompanies degenerative disk disease with joint-margin spurring and joint hypertrophy (Mooney & Robertson, 1976). The worker should use joint-protection techniques to avoid twisting and joint compression in extremely lordotic postures, particularly when lifting a load.

In the rehabilitation of an injured worker, the therapist must constantly find the balance between immobilization and mobilization to promote healing of injured tissues and maintain function. Progressive functional activities must be introduced in accordance with the severity of the injury, the condition of the tissues, and the time elapsed in the healing process.

The following guidelines can be used to ensure successful rehabilitation and functional training after lifting injuries:

1. Specific muscle strengthening and reconditioning of the trunk, hip extensor, and quadriceps muscles should be used to protect the spinal ligaments, joints, and disks.
2. Protective and supported progressive loading should be considered in ligamentous injuries to promote healing and prevent chronic instability.
3. Progressive loading of the spine with increasing weight, frequency, and duration of lifting should be carefully monitored for symptoms and recovery if the worker has degenerative disk disease.
4. Protective posturing and lifting techniques should be determined for degenerative joint disease, spondylosis, and foraminal stenosis.
5. General cardiovascular and muscular reconditioning should be undertaken, particularly if the worker engages in high-frequency lifting of long duration.

The goal is to minimize compressive forces, avoid torsional and tensile stresses, avoid extremes of flexion and extension, and adopt protective and adaptive body mechanics based on the individual needs of the injured worker.

Environmental Conditions

Lighting should provide visual support for perception of depth and surface texture. Temperature should be within the comfort zone of 65 to 70°F. Proper coupling between the work surfaces and the feet should meet the recommended coefficient of friction of .4 to .5 by providing a level, dry, nonslippery work surface (see Chapter 5 for a discussion of environmental design). The style, sole, and heel of work shoes should be appropriate to allow flexibility and protection from slipping. Clothing should allow full flexibility, comfort, and contact with objects (NIOSH, 1981).

Lift Testing and Analysis

Lift testing should provide the most information about the readiness or ability of a worker to perform the specific lifting task. The problem with lift testing with standardized machines or protocols is the poor translation to performance of the actual task in the workplace. When considering a testing method, one should ask the following questions:

- Does the test measure what it is supposed to measure?
- Is the test reliable?
- Can the test be rated against standardized norms?
- Can the test be rated against itself?
- Is the test safe?
- Is the test effective in identifying workers at risk for injury?
- Is the test suitable for administration by trained nonmedical personnel? (Gagnon & Smyth, 1992; Keyserling et al, 1980)

The four methods of lift testing most widely used are static (isometric), isokinetic, isoinertial, and psychophysical. Static testing measures isometric strength in a defined range of motion with a constrained posture (Mayer et al, 1988a). Isokinetic testing measures torque about a fixed axis with constant speed and variable force through defined ranges of motion and semiconstrained postures (Sapega, 1990). Isoinertial testing measures a person's ability to move a constant force with variable speeds through defined ranges of motion with unconstrained postures (Mayer et al, 1988a). Psychophysical testing measures the subjective perception of acceptable weight or effort in dynamic or static conditions (Snook, 1978). Each method has advantages and disadvantages to be considered when choosing a testing method to evaluate lifting ability.

Static Lifting Tests

Static (isometric) lifting tests usually require a minimum of three maximal-effort isometric lifting efforts in the position of the pick-up phase of the lift. The test design has high test-retest reliability (Chaffin & Park, 1973; Zeh et al, 1986). It provides for controlled exertion, but studies have indicated that use of some testing positions have resulted in injuries (Zeh et al, 1986). The predictive value for risk for injury on the job is poor (NIOSH, 1981). The static strength value must exceed the weight of the object to be lifted dynamically to allow for the acceleration effects at pick-up. Static testing does not test the handling and strength requirements of the transfer and placement phases of the lift. The biomechanical stresses of a dynamic lift increase 15 to 20% above those of a static lift (Chaffin & Park, 1973; Keyserling et al, 1980; Pytel & Kamon, 1981). There is poor correlation between the maximum acceptable dynamic weight value and the maximum voluntary contraction value obtained with static testing.

Isokinetic Lifting Test

Isokinetic testing requires several repetitions of the required arc or motion at various speeds. The test design has high test-retest reliability. It provides for controlled exertion. There have been no known injuries with this testing method. The predictive value for risk for injury on the job is poor. The isokinetic value does not correlate with the dynamic strength value because lifting does not occur with constant speed and variable force. In addition, endurance testing with isokinetic tests has low test-retest reliability and poor correlation with functional performance (Noe et al, 1990; Sapega, 1990).

Isoinertial Lifting Tests

Isoinertial testing requires the completion of a dynamic task in which an object is picked up and lifted vertically or through an arc of motion. Isoinertial testing most accurately simulates the actual lifting task. Acceleration is included in the testing. If placement of the object is part of the test design, deceleration forces are also included. Isoinertial vertical lifting loses the trajectory of motion and the deceleration forces of the actual lift. The most important disadvantages of isoinertial testing are subjectivity and the possibility of observer and measurement errors (Mayer et al, 1988a; 1988b).

Psychophysical Lifting Tests

Psychophysical testing requires a subjective measurement of acceptance by the lifter of the maximum value of weight or rate of work for a given lifting task. There is a high correlation between perceived acceptable limits and physiologic parameters of fatigue (Hogan & Fleishman, 1979; NIOSH, 1981; Snook, 1978). The risk for back injury is three times greater in jobs that are perceived as unacceptable by more than 25% of the population (Snook, 1978). Psychophysical testing with both dynamic and static testing methods has been used to determine that the maximum acceptable isometric value is the second lowest. In performance of maximum effort, the isometric value with static testing is the highest value and the dynamic value with isoinertial testing is second highest.

Measuring perceived effort of a lifting task is one way to measure acceptance of a load. A perceived-effort scale based on the Borg Relative Perceived Effort Scale has been developed and validated for occupational tasks (Hogan, 1980). Perceived effort is rated on a graded scale from 1 to 7. Each number corresponds to a verbal description as follows:

1. Very, very light
2. Very light
3. Light
4. Somewhat hard
5. Hard

6. Very hard
7. Very, very hard

The scale may be useful in a progressive lifting test and to correlate perceived effort with increasing workload in a work-hardening program.

Designing a Lifting Test

The best test incorporates the important aspects of lifting and represents the true dynamic nature of the lifting task. The test should be safe and easy to administer. Scoring methods should have minimal observer error and should incorporate psychophysical testing, especially in the determination of risk for injury or reinjury at work. Considerations in the design of a lifting test should address the following important aspects of lifting ability:

- Adequate muscle flexibility and joint mobility to perform the task through the required range of motion
- Adequate strength to lift the object through the required range of motion
- Control of the object in pick-up, transfer, and placement that correlates with concentric and eccentric muscle control
- Appropriate handling behaviors of proper postural orientation, base of support, foot positioning, and pivoting
- Perceived effort scores of acceptance of weight equal to or less than the maximum acceptable weight or maximum acceptable rate of lifting
- No increase in pain or other symptoms during the lift and after the lifting period
- Adequate recovery time to be able to repeat the same performance at a specified rate with the same values without undue soreness, stiffness, or pain
- Acceptable predetermined individual values for physiologic responses of heart rate, blood pressure, and muscle fatigue.

Lifting tests designed and validated with healthy subjects should not be used for determining lifting capabilities for injured workers. The best method for testing the lifting capability of an injured worker considers safety first and closely simulates the actual lifting task.

Conclusion

Lifting injuries can be accidental, overexertional, or cumulative. Cost-effective injury prevention and management should include strategies based on the cause of the injury. Injury prevention includes screening, lifting design, and training and education. Many factors are important in determining the safety of the lifting task. NIOSH standards have been revised to include symmetric lifting in addition to size, weight, horizontal distance, vertical location, vertical distance, and frequency and duration of the lifting task. The standards apply to the safety limits of an uninjured worker. Age limits must be considered for a previously injured worker. Residual impairments and the pathologic condition of the tissues may alter the responses to the demands of lifting and require modification of the biomechanics or variables of the task.

Functional rehabilitation specific to the lifting task requires knowledge of the variables of the task and knowledge of the physical, behavioral, and psychologic limitations of the injured worker. Successful return to safe lifting requires education and training of the worker and possibly a modification of the lifting task.

References

Adams, M.A., Hutton W.C. (1982). Prolapsed intervertebral disc: A hyperflexion injury. Spine, 7:184-191.

Andersson, G.B.J., Ortengren R., Nachemson, A. (1976). Quantitative studies of back loads in lifting. Spine, 1:178-185.

Batti'e, M.C., Bigos, S.J., Fisher, L.D., et al (1989a). A prospective study of the role of cardiovascular risk factors and fitness in industrial back pain complaints. Spine, 14:141-147.

Batti'e, M.C., Bigos, S.J., Fisher, L.D., et al (1989b). Isometric lifting strength as a predictor of industrial back pain reports. Spine, 14:851-856.

Bejjani, F.J., Gross, C.M., Pugh, J.W. (1984). Model for static lifting: Relationship of loads on the spine and the knee. Journal of Biomechanics, 17:281-286.

Blankenship, K.L., Blankenship, L.S. (1986). Lifting Guide. Ohio: American Therapeutics.

Chaffin, D.B., Park, K.S. (1973). A longitudinal study of low back pain as associated with occupational weight lifting factors. American Industrial Hygiene Association Journal, 34:513-524.

Dempster, W.T. (1955). Space Requirements of the Seated Operator. Ohio, Wright-Patterson Air Force Base (WADCTR 55-159).

Drury, C.G., Law, C., Pawenski, C.S. (1982). A survey of industrial box handling. Human Factors, 24:553-565.

Elling, R. (1989). The political economy of workers' health and safety. Social Science and Medicine, 28:1171-1182.

Farfan, H.F. (1970). The effects of torsion on the lumbar intervertebral joints: The role of torsion in the production of disc degeneration. Journal of Bone and Joint Surgery, 52:468-483.

Gagnon, M., Smyth, G. (1992). Biomechanical exploration on dynamic modes of lifting. Ergonomics, 35:329-345.

Gordon, S.J., Yang, K.H., Mayer, P.J., Mace, A.H., Kish, V.L., Radin, E.L. (1990). Mechanism of disc rupture. Spine, 16:450-456.

Gracovetsky, S., Kary, M., Levy, S., Sen Siad, R., Pitchen, I., Helie, J. (1990). Analysis of spinal and muscular activity during flexion/extension and free lifts. Spine, 15:1333-1339.

Hampton, D., Laros, G., McCarron, R., Franks, D. (1989). Healing potential of the anulus fibrosus. Spine, 14:398-401.

Hebert, L., Miller, G. (1987). Newer heavy load lifting methods help firms reduce back injuries. Occupational Health and Safety, 2:57-60.

Hogan, J.C. (1980). The state of the art of strength testing. In D.C. Walsh, R.H. Egdahl (Eds.), Women, Work, and Health: Challenges to Corporate Policy. New York: Springer-Verlag.

Hogan, J.C., Fleishman, E.A. (1979). An index of the physical effort required in human task performance. Journal of Applied Psychology, 64:197-204.

Jiang, B.C., Ayoub, M.M. (1987). Modelling of maximum acceptable load of lifting by physical factors. Ergonomics, 30:529-538.

Kazarian, L.E. (1975). Creep characteristics of the human spinal column. Orthopedic Clinics of North America, 6:3-18.

Keyserling, W.M., Herrin, G.D., Chaffin, D.B., Armstrong, T.J., Foss, M.L. (1980). Establishing an industrial strength testing program. American Industrial Hygiene Association Journal, 41:730-736.

Kumar, S. (1984). The physiological cost of three different methods of lifting in sagittal and lateral planes. Ergonomics, 27:425-433.

Kumar, S., Davis, P.R. (1983). Spinal loading in static and dynamic postures: EMG and intra-abdominal pressure study. Ergonomics, 26: 913-926.

Liles, D.H., Mahajan, P. (1985). Using NIOSH lifting guide decreases risks of back injuries. Occupational Health and Safety, 57-60.

Matheson, L.N., Ogden, L.D. (1983). Work Tolerance Screening. Trabuco Canyon: Rehabilitation Institute of Southern California.

Mayer, T.G., Barnes, D., Kishino, N.D., et al (1988a). Progressive isoinertial lifting evaluation. 1. A standardized protocol and normative database. Spine, 13:993-997.

Mayer, T.H., Barnes, D., Nichols, G., et al (1988b). Progressive isoinertial lifting evaluation. 2. A comparison with isokinetic lifting in a disabled chronic low-back pain industrial population. Spine, 13:998-1002.

McGill, S.M., Norman, R.W. (1986). Partitioning of the L4-L5 dynamic moment into disc, ligamentous and muscular components during lifting. Spine, 11:666-678.

Mooney, V., Robertson, J. (1976). The facet syndrome. Clinical Orthopedics and Related Research, 115:149-156.

National Institute for Occupational Safety and Health [NIOSH] (1981). Work Practices Guide for Manual Lifting. Technical Report 81-122. Cincinnati: NIOSH Division of Biomedical and Behavioral Science.

Nicholson, L.M., Legg, S.J. (1986). A psychophysical study of the effects of load and frequency upon selection of workload in repetitive lifting. Ergonomics, 29:903-911.

Noe, D.A., Mostardi, R.A., Jackson, M.E., Porterfield, J.A., Askew, M.J. (1990). Myoelectric activity and sequencing of selected trunk muscles during isokinetic lifting. Spine, 17:225-229.

Noone. G., Mazumdar, J. (1992). Lifting low-lying loads in sagittal plane. Ergonomics, 35:65-92.

Patterson, P., Congleton, J., Koppa, R., Huchingson, R.D. (1987). The effects of load knowledge on stresses at the lower back during lifting. Ergonomics, 30:539-549.

Pheasant, S. (1991). Ergonomics, Work and Health. Gaithersburg, Md.: Aspen.

Pope, M.H. (1987). The biomechanical basis for early care programmes. Ergonomics, 30:351-358.

Putz-Anderson, V., Waters, T. (1991). Revisions in NIOSH Guide to Manual Lifting. Presented to the National Conference for a National Strategy for Occupational Musculoskeletal Injury Prevention: Implementation Issues and Research Needs, Ann Arbor.

Pytel, J.L., Kamon, E. (1981). Dynamic strength test as a predictor for maximal and acceptable lifting. Ergonomics, 24:663-672.

Sapega, A.A. (1990). Current concepts review of muscle performance evaluation in orthopaedic practice. Journal of Bone and Joint Surgery, 72:1562-1574.

Snook, S.H. (1978). The design of manual handling tasks. Ergonomics, 21:963-985.

Snook, S.H., White, A.H. (1984). Education and training. In M.H. Pope, J.W. Frymoyer, G. Andersson (Eds.), Occupational Low Back Pain. New York: Praeger.

Tichauer, E.R. (1971). A pilot study of the biomechanics of lifting in simulated industrial work situations. Journal of Safety Research, 3:98-115.

Troup, J.D.G. (1977). Dynamic factors in the analysis of stoop and crouch lifting methods: A methodological approach to the development of safe materials handling standards. Orthopedic Clinics of North America, 8:201-209.

Waikar, A., Lee, K., Aghazadeh, F., Parks, C. (1991). Evaluating lifting tasks using subjective and biomechanical estimates of stress at the lower back. Ergonomics, 34:33-47.

Zeh, J., Hansson, T., Bigos, S., Spengler, D., Batti'e, M., Wortley, M. (1986). Isometric strength testing recommendations based on a statistical analysis of the procedure. Spine, 11:43-46.

CHAPTER 8

Revised 1991 NIOSH Equation for the Design and Evaluation of Manual Lifting Tasks

Diane Aja

ABSTRACT

The 1981 lift formula published by the National Institute of Occupational Safety and Health (NIOSH) has been revised on the basis of research and recommendations from health care providers and ergonomic specialists. The new formula changes some of the original criteria and includes a way to allow for asymmetric lifting and coupling.

In 1985, the prevention of work-related injuries to the lower part of the back was identified by a scientific review panel as a goal to be included in the *Proposed National Strategy for the Prevention of Work Related Musculoskeletal Injuries* (1986). This document serves as a blueprint for musculoskeletal research at the National Institute for Occupational Safety and Health (NIOSH). Consensus at the time was that despite changes in the engineering and design of work sites, employee training in lifting techniques, and worker placement and evaluation, the rate of injuries continues to increase. A report entitled *Back Injuries* published in 1982 by the United States Department of Labor Bureau of Labor and Statistics provided the following data:

- Back injuries account for nearly 20% of all injuries and illnesses in the workplace
- Back injuries account for nearly 25% of annual worker compensation payments

A 1988 report by the National Safety Council entitled *Accident Facts* revealed the following:

- Overexertion is the most common cause of occupational injury, approaching 31% of all injuries
- The back is the body part most frequently injured—22% of 1.7 million injuries

After 15 years of research on work-related low-back pain and manual lifting, the following three concepts are generally accepted:

1. Many workers who perform manual lifting are at risk for injuries to the lower part of the back.
2. If the task exceeds the worker's physical capacity, low-back pain is likely to occur.
3. Workers who perform the same job show great variation in their physical strengths and limitations (Waters et al, 1993).

Work Practices Guide 1981

In 1981, NIOSH published the *Work Practices Guide for Manual Lifting*. This document demonstrated that NIOSH recognized the growing problem of work-related back injuries. The *Work Practices Guide* proposed that when job demands exceed worker capabilities, overexertion injuries occur. The theory of overexertion injury led to the conceptualization of the following lifting model:

$$\text{Strain index (SI)} = \text{Job demands} / \text{Worker capacity}$$

Under ideal work conditions SI ≤ 1.0, which indicates that worker capacities are greater than or equal to job demands. The risk for overexertion injury increases as job demands exceed worker abilities (SI > 1.0). A simple example of the strain index is a job that requires a 70-pound (32-kg) lifting standard. If a worker can lift only 35 pounds (16 kg) comfortably, SI = 70/35 = 2, indicating a high risk for overexertion injury.

The *Work Practices Guide for Manual Lifting* reviewed the lifting-related research through 1981 and presented recommendations to control risks associated with manual materials-lifting jobs. An equation was introduced that allowed calculation of the recommended weight in the performance of a symmetric, two-handed lifting task. In addition to these characteristics, the lifting task needed to be smooth with good coupling, unrestricted lifting posture, and favorable ambient conditions, and the width of the object lifted could not not be more than 30 inches (76.2 cm). Two parameters were calculated with the formula—the action limit (AL) and the maximum permissible limit (MPL). The AL was defined as the estimated average weight of lift for a given job that could be safely handled by 99% of the male working population and 75% of the female working population. It was the recommended weight derived from the lifting equation. The MPL was the AL multiplied by three (NIOSH, 1981).

After the lifting equation was applied to the lifting task, the actual weight of the object being lifted was compared to the AL and the MPL. In situations in which the lifting task was greater than the MPL, the lifting task was deemed unacceptable without engineering redesign. If the AL was less than the lifting task and the lifting task was less than the MPL, the lift would be deemed unacceptable without administrative or engineering controls. Administrative controls included worker selection and training to decrease the risks associated with hazardous lifting. Engineering controls included ergonomic modifications of the workplace to enhance worker safety. Lifting tasks calculated to be less than the AL represented nominal risk to most industrial work forces. Figure 8–1 compares the MPL and AL in relation to weight lifted and horizontal location of the load.

The specific lifting equation as outlined in the 1981 *Work Practices Guide for Manual Lifting* was as follows

$$AL = 90 \times (6 / H) \times [1 - (.01 \ |V - 30|)] \times [.7 + (3 / D)] \times [1 - (F / F_{max})]$$
(U.S. Customary)

$$AL = 40 \times (15/H) \times (1 \ .004 \ |V - 75|) \times [.7 + (7.5/D)] \times [1 - (F/F_{max})]$$
(metric)

where H is the horizontal distance of the load from the worker; V, the vertical distance of the load at the beginning of the lift; D, the distance traveled during the lift; F, the frequency of lifting; and F_{max}, the frequency coefficient based on a 1- or 8-hour day. (The frequency coefficient is derived from a table.)

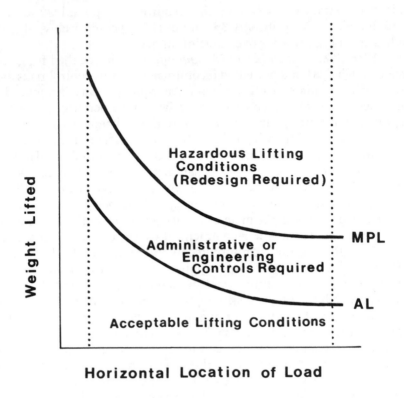

Figure 8–1   Weight in relation to horizontal location of the load during a lift. (NIOSH, 1981)

Revised Lifting Equation

Impetus for Revising the Lifting Equation

The first 4 years after the introduction of the 1981 NIOSH lift formula brought criticism that was both positive and negative. Health care providers and safety specialists, who were pleased to finally have an objective way to evaluate lifting jobs for the purposes of reducing risk of injuries in industry, praised the formula. In a field study designed to test the validity and applicability of the NIOSH formula, data on 101 different lifting jobs were collected over a period of several years. The authors used the AL method to identify jobs that were causing problems in terms of injury rate and higher cost of medical and wage compensation when an injury did occur. The authors concluded that "the NIOSH method has a high potential for reducing the incidence and severity of manual materials handling injury" (Liles and Mahajan, 1985, p. 60).

What frustrated investigators who tried to use the 1981 formula was the way lifting tasks were defined for application purposes. Few industrial settings incorporate symmetric, two-handed lifting in the sagittal plane with good hand-to-object coupling. On the contrary, most industrial lifting tasks are asymmetric in nature, the load being lifted at the side of the body. Mitral and Fard (1986) investigated the effects of symmetric and asymmetric lifting on the maximum lifting ability and physiologic effort. Results with 18 young male subjects indicated that the subjects reduced their acceptable lifting weight by approximately 8.5% when they lifted asymmetrically. In addition, lower maximum acceptable weights were lifted when the loads were lifted asymmetrically. The subjects stated that asymmetric lifting was more physically stressful than symmetric lifting and, thus, was not their preference when performing lifting tasks. From a physiologic perspective, negligible differences in oxygen uptake or heart rate could be detected when subjects lifted asymmetrically as opposed to symmetrically.

As stated previously, variations in hand-to-object coupling could not be incorporated into the 1981 formula. The reality of most industrial settings is that good hand-to-object coupling is rare. Since 1980, Drury et al have been investigating the role of hand placement and characteristics in box-handling tasks. The results of a 1989 study revealed that having no handles was the worst scenario in symmetric lifting and lowering. Handles near the top center of the box were most helpful in floor-to-waist lifting. In loading and unloading pallets, in which all heights are involved, the ideal handle location varied according to the weight of the object being moved (Drury et al, 1989).

Procedures Used to Develop the Revision

In 1985, a panel of experts and experienced users were asked to review the *Work Practices Guide for Manual Lifting* (1981) and to identify background data for the revision. Five public meetings were held between 1987 and 1990 in which the following questions were discussed:

- Do the existing methods and the equation provided in the *Work Practices Guide* yield a realistic assessment of the potential for overexertion injury in two-handed repetitive lifts in the sagittal plane?
- Can asymmetric lifting tasks be explained by expanding the 1981 formula?
- Can new data on manual lifting hazards be reflected in a revision of the 1981 formula? (Putz-Anderson & Waters, 1991)

A three-step process was undertaken to revise the 1981 method and equation to answer these questions. The first step involved an extensive review of the lifting literature since 1981. The literature search revealed that factors limiting a worker's ability to lift include the worker's strength, maximum disk compression, cardiovascular capacity, and perceived lifting discomfort. The following four reports were compiled to summarize the research on the physiologic, biomechanical, psychophysical, and epidemiologic aspects of lifting:

- Physiological Basis for Manual Lifting Guidelines (Rodgers & Yates, 1991)
- Biomechanical Basis for Manual Lifting Guidelines (Garg, 1991a)
- Psychophysical Basis for Manual Lifting Guidelines (Ayoub, 1991)
- Epidemiological Basis for Manual Lifting Guidelines (Garg, 1991b)

The second step of the formula revision process involved identifying research articles that contained key data on lifting limitations when the load varied in horizontal and vertical displacements. Some of the more well-defined studies had subjects perform lifting activities while varying frequency and duration. From these data, summary tables of acceptable load weights for specified population percentiles were tabulated (Garg & Badger, 1986; Garg, 1989;, Batti'e et al, 1989; Ruhmann & Schmidtke, 1989; Snook & Ciriello, 1991).

The third step of the revision of the lifting formula involved developing the three critical technical components of the lifting equation: the standard lifting location (SLL), the load constant (LC), and the multipliers or coefficients that represent the task factors. The SLL provides a three-dimensional reference point to characterize a worker's lifting posture. The SLL for the 1981 formula was defined as a vertical height of 30 inches (76 cm) and a horizontal distance of 6 inches (15 cm), as measured from the midpoint between the ankles. Studies such as that performed by Rhumann and Schmidtke (1989) supported an ideal vertical lifting height of 30 inches (76 cm), but the 6-inch (15-cm) horizontal distance was disputed. Garg (1989) used a laboratory study to compare the actual lifting ability of male college students with those calculated with the NIOSH lifting formula. He also compared the MPLs based on measured horizontal distances with those based on guideline recommendations:

$$H = [6 + \left(\frac{W}{2}\right)] \text{ inches}$$

where H is the horizontal distance and W is the distance of the load away from the body measured in the horizontal axis (Figure 8–2).

The results showed that the measured horizontal distance was much greater than the horizontal distance generated by the formula in the 1981 NIOSH lifting guidelines. This research and that of others supported increasing the horizontal factor from 6 inches (15 cm) to 10 inches (25 cm). Workers tend to hold objects farther away from the body than originally believed; the revised formula protects them with an increased horizontal factor.

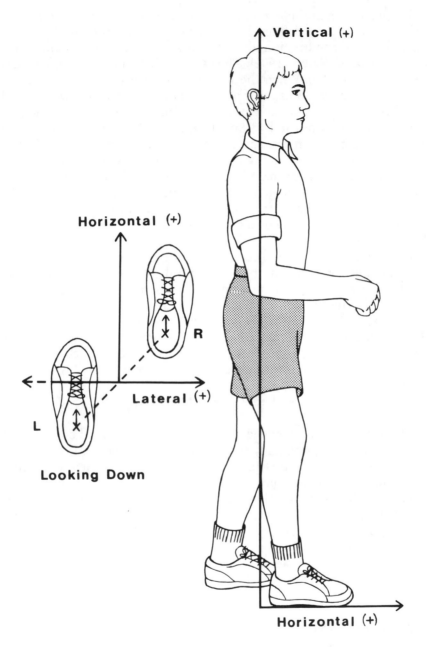

Figure 8–2 Vertical, lateral, and horizontal axes. (From NIOSH, 1991.)

The second critical component of the equation evaluated by the panel was the LC. The LC is defined as the maximum weight value for the SLL, based on selected conditions and constraints associated with manual lifting (Putz-Anderson & Waters, 1991). The LC established for the 1981 equation was 90 pounds (41 kg). When the lifting formula was revised, the LC was reduced to 51 pounds (23 kg). Part of the need to lower the LC was related to the increase in the horizontal factor from 6 inches (15 cm) to 10 inches (25 cm). In addition, new research by Snook and Ciriello (1991) revealed that the maximum acceptable lifting capacity of female workers was less than estimated when the 1981 formula was developed. The revised LC of 51 pounds (23 kg), combined with optimal SLL conditions such as no twisting and good coupling, would be acceptable to 75% of female workers and 99% of male workers. By lowering the LC from 90 pounds (41 kg) to 51 pounds (23 kg), the revised formula should provide a greater degree of protection for the industrial work force.

The revised lifting equation contains multipliers or coefficients similar to the task variables presented in the 1981 formula. There are six multipliers in the 1991 lifting formula. They represent the horizontal, vertical, distance, asymmetric, frequency, and coupling factors involved in the actual task of lifting. The role of the multipliers is to reduce the maximum weight value of the LC to compensate for lifting conditions that are not ideal. Each multiplier can vary from 1.0 for optimal lifting conditions to 0.0 for high-strain lifting conditions. The 1991 lifting formula can be described in the following way:

$$RWL = LC \times HM \times VM \times DM \times AM \times FM \times CM$$

where RWL is the recommended weight limit; LC, the load constant; HM, the horizontal multiplier; VM, the vertical multiplier; DM, the distance multiplier; AM, the asymmetric multiplier; FM, the frequency multiplier; and CM, the coupling multiplier.

The research that the led to the development of each multiplier can be found in the following publications: horizontal (Snook & Ciriello, 1991; Garg et al, 1983); vertical (Snook & Ciriello, 1991; Punnett et al, 1987); distance (Garg et al, 1978; Snook & Ciriello, 1991); asymmetry (Garg & Badger, 1986; Garg & Banaag, 1988); frequency (Garg et al, 1978); coupling (Garg & Saxena, 1980; Smith & Jiang, 1984).

Comparison of 1981 and 1991 Formulas

Similarities

The first similarity is that research data in the areas of biomechanics, work physiology, psychophysics, and epidemiology were used when both formulas were developed. Second, both equations allow the lift to be broken into task

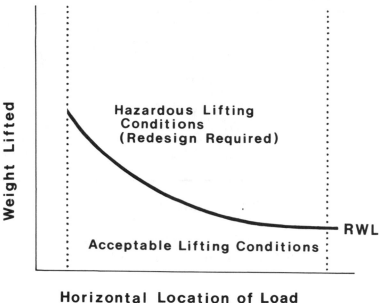

Horizontal Location of Load

Figure 8–3   Weight lifted in relation to horizontal location of load during lifting. (From Putz-Anderson & Waters, 1991.)

variables that can be altered for a safe lift. In addition, a safe lift can be calculated from both versions using a multiplicative lifting equation. A multiplicative lifting equation allows for interaction between a variety of task factors (eg, horizontal distance, lifting frequency) while imposing a uniform set of mathematical rules to regulate the influence of the task factors. Last, both equations provide a zone of acceptable lifting strain above which engineering or other interventions should be applied. Figure 8–3 is a graph of the cut-off zone for the 1991 equation, which can be compared with the 1981 cut-off zone in Figure 8–1 (Putz-Anderson & Waters, 1991).

Differences

The differences between the two equations are presented in Table 8–1. Two important differences are apparent. The first is that the 1991 formula contains two additional task factors: asymmetry and hand-container coupling. The second difference is that the 1991 formula provides one recommended weight limit (RWL), whereas the 1981 formula provided two (AL and MPL).

Table 8–1 Comparison of Lifting Equations

Factor	Multiplier (Value)	
	1981	*1991*
Load Constant	90 pounds	51 pounds
Horizontal	6/H	10/H
Vertical	$1-(.01 |V-30|)$	$1-(.0075 |V-30|)$
Distance	.7 + 3/D	.82 + 1.8/D
Frequency	$1 - F/F_{max}$	from table
Asymmetry	not available	1 – .0032A
Coupling	not available	from table

Implementation of the 1991 Equation

$$\text{RWL} = 51 \text{ lbs} \times (10/H) \times [1-(.0075 |V-30|)] \times [.82 + (1.8/D)] \times (1 - .0032A)$$
$$\times (\text{FM from table}) \times (\text{CM from table})$$
(U.S. Customary)

$$\text{RWL} = 23 \text{ kg} \times (25/H) \times [1 - (.003 |V - 75|)] \times [.82 + (4.5/D)] \times (1 - .0032A)$$
$$\times (\text{FM from table}) \times (\text{CM from table})$$
(metric)

H is the horizontal distance of the hands from the midpoint between the ankles. It is measured (in inches) from the midpoint of the line that joins the ankles to the midpoint at which the hands grasp the object while in the lifting position at the origin and destination of the lift (Figure 8–2).

V is the vertical distance of the hands from the floor. The distance is measured from the floor to the point at which the hands grasp the object at the origin and the destination of the lift (Figure 8–2).

D is the vertical travel distance between the origin and the destination of the lift. V origin is subtracted from V destination to obtain D. Take the absolute value if D is a negative number.

A is the angle of asymmetry, the angular displacement of the load from the sagittal plane. A plumb line is dropped to the floor at the beginning of the lift. The examiner uses the plumb line to draw in chalk on the floor the direction of the lift at the origin and the destination of the lift. Cardboard X's also can be used to mark the plumb-line measurements. A goniometer is used to measure in degrees the angle of asymmetry (Figure 8–4). For a given weight, asymmetric lifting is more likely to cause injury and should be replaced by symmetric lifting whenever possible.

FM, the frequency multiplier, is the average frequency of lifting measured in lifts per minute and determined by the frequency and duration of the lift. The duration of the lift is defined as short, moderate, or long. For a

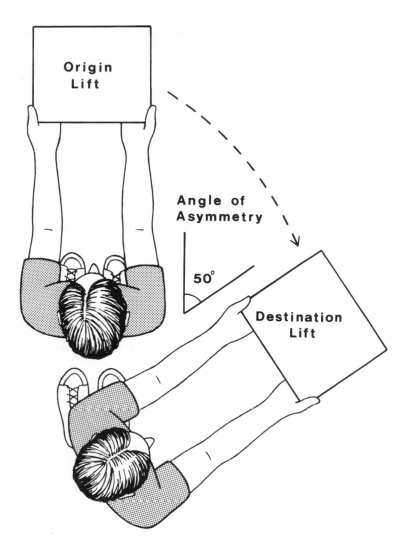

Origin Lift

Angle of Asymmetry

50°

Destination Lift

Figure 8–4   Overhead view of asymmetric lift.

lift to be classified as short in duration, lifting is continuous for as long as 1 hour followed by a recovery period of at least 120% of work time. For example, if an employee lifts for 30 minutes, at least the next 36 minutes should be spent in nonlifting work. Moderate lifting is defined as continuous lifting for up to 2 hours followed by a recovery period of at least 30% of work time. For example, if an employee lifts for 2 hours, nonlifting work activities should be performed for at least 36 minutes. Lifting of long duration is lifting up to 8 hours with no additional fatigue allowances other than normal breaks.

Table 8-2 Frequency Multiplier (FM) Table

Frequency	Work Duration (Continuous)					
	≤ 8 Hours		*≤ 2 Hours*		*≤ 1 Hour*	
Lifts/Min	V < 30	V ≥ 30	V < 30	V ≥ 30	V < 30	V ≥ 30
0.2	0.85	0.85	0.95	0.95	1.00	1.00
0.5	0.81	0.81	0.92	0.92	0.97	0.97
1	0.75	0.75	0.88	0.88	0.94	0.94
2	0.65	0.65	0.84	0.84	0.91	0.91
3	0.55	0.55	0.79	0.79	0.88	0.88
4	0.45	0.45	0.72	0.72	0.84	0.84
5	0.35	0.35	0.60	0.60	0.80	0.80
6	0.27	0.27	0.50	0.50	0.75	0.75
7	0.22	0.22	0.42	0.42	0.70	0.70
8	0.18	0.18	0.35	0.35	0.60	0.60
9	0.00	0.15	0.30	0.30	0.52	0.52
10	0.00	0.13	0.26	0.26	0.45	0.45
11	0.00	0.00	0.00	0.23	0.41	0.41
12	0.00	0.00	0.00	0.21	0.37	0.37
13	0.00	0.00	0.00	0.00	0.00	0.34
14	0.00	0.00	0.00	0.00	0.00	0.31
15	0.00	0.00	0.00	0.00	0.00	0.28
>15	0.00	0.00	0.00	0.00	0.00	0.00

Values of vertical height (V) are in inches. To convert inches to centimeters multiply by 254 and divide by 100. (Source: Putz-Anderson & Waters, 1991)

For Table 8–2 to be used accurately, all criteria used to determine the frequency and duration of the lift must be met.

CM is the coupling multiplier. Table 8–3 is used to establish the coupling multiplier. The maximum force a worker can exert on an object is greatly affected by the nature of hand-to-object coupling. Good coupling can reduce the maximum grasp forces required and increase acceptable lifting weight. Poor coupling requires higher grasp forces and decreases the acceptable lifting weight. Because lifting is a dynamic process, the quality of hand-to-object coupling may vary throughout the lift. An average has to be taken to establish the overall effectiveness of coupling during the entire lift. If there is any doubt about how to classify a particular coupling design, the most stressful classification should be selected.

Table 8–3 Coupling Multiplier

Couplings	V < 30 inches	V ≥ 30 inches
Good	1.00	1.00
Fair	.95	1.00
Poor	.90	.90

V = vertical height; 30 inches = 76 cm.

Good Coupling

- Handles are designed to be 0.75-1.5 inches (2-4 cm) in diameter, more than 4.5 inches (11 cm) long, have 2 inches (5 cm) of clearance, a cylindrical shape, and a smooth, nonslip surface
- Handhold cutouts are 3 inches (8 cm) high, 4.5 inches (11 cm) long, semioval, have 2 inches (5 cm) of clearance, and a smooth, nonslip surface. The container must be 0.43 inch (1 cm) or more thick
- Container is 16 inches (41 cm) or longer in front, 12 inches (30 cm) or less high, and has a smooth, nonslip surface
- If the load is not boxed, the worker can comfortably wrap a hand around the object with no wrist deviation, no awkward postures, and no excessive force in the grip

Fair Coupling

- Handles or handhold cut-outs at less than optimal design
- A worker is able to clamp the fingers at nearly 90 degrees under the container if there are no handles or cut-outs

Poor Coupling

- Container is 16 inches (41 cm) or longer in front, 12 inches (30 cm) or more high, has a rough or slippery surface, sharp edges, an asymmetric center of mass, unstable contents, or requires use of gloves

- Container has no handles or cut-outs

Figure 8–5 can be used to classify the coupling multiplier.

Limitations of the 1991 Lifting Equation

The 1991 lifting formula is applicable only to lifting tasks that fit the following conditions:

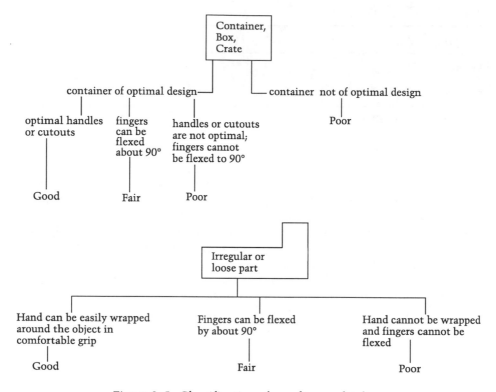

Figure 8–5   Classification of coupling multiplier.

1. Work environment has a favorable temperature, such as 65-80°F (18-27°C) and no more than 50% humidity
2. Other work tasks do not require a high expenditure of energy
3. The lifting task is two-handed and is not performed in a high-speed, jerky manner
4. The worker-floor surface coupling has friction that is similar to that between a smooth, dry floor and the sole of a clean, dry leather work shoe.

Lifting Index

The lifting index (LI) provides a simple estimate of the hazard of overexertion injury for a manual lifting job. The use of a single number for report-writing may be useful for therapists when they share information with industrial workers. Long mathematical formulas and calculations may be confusing and intimidating as well as time-consuming to read. The LI can be used as a relative measure of job severity and can help companies with numerous ergonomic problems decide which to address first. In addition, industry can focus on a long-term lifting problem by using the LI to break the problem into short-term goals. For example, if the LI for a specific lifting task is 4.0, the short-term goal could be reducing that number to 3.0 with a long-term goal of reaching 1.0 or less.

$$LI = \frac{L}{RWL}$$

where L is the weight of the object being lifted and RWL is the number calculated in the 1991 lifting formula. If LI > 1.0, overexertion injury is likely because job demands exceed recommended weight. If LI < 1.0, the job presents minimal risk for overexertion injury.

Case Study 1

Job Description

Harold works as a cook and order-taker at a fast-food restaurant. He is 6 feet, 4 inches (193 cm) tall, of slender build, and the primary provider for his family. After suffering sporadic low-back pain for several years, Harold received the diagnosis of "acquired spinal stenosis with right shooting leg pain." Harold experiences the most pain when he repetitively hands trays of food to customers during a busy lunch hour. The counter is 36 inches (91 cm) wide, 48 inches (122 cm) high at the customer service end, and 36 inches (91 cm) high where the worker fills the trays with food. The filled trays of food weigh as much as 5 pounds (2.3 kg), and the worker is not allowed to slide the tray of food across the counter.

Job Analysis

The calculations using the 1981 formula are as follows:

$$AL = 90 \times (6 / H) \times [1 - (.01 |V- 30|)] \times [.7 + (3 / D)] \times [1- (F / F_{max})]$$

H origin = 18 inches (46 cm)	V origin = 42 inches (107 cm)
H destination = 30 inches (76 cm)	V destination = 50 inches (127 cm)
D = 8 inches (20 cm)	F = 4 lifts per minute

$$F_{max} = 18 \text{ (from } F_{max} \text{ table, NIOSH, 1981)}$$

$$\text{AL (destination)} = 90 \times (6/30) \times [1 - (.01\ |50 - 30|)] \times [.7 + (3/8)]$$
$$\times [1 - (4/18)]$$

$$= 90 \times .2 \times .8 \times 1.075 \times .78$$

$$= 12 \text{ pounds } (5.4 \text{ kg})$$

The calculations using the 1991 lifting formula are as follows:

$$\text{RWL (destination)} = 51 \times (10/H) \times [1 - (.0075\ |V - 30|)] \times [.82 + (1.8/D)]$$
$$\times (1 - .0032A) \times FM \times CM$$

H origin = 18 inches (46 cm)	V origin = 30 inches (76 cm)
H destination = 30 inches (76 cm)	V destination = 50 inches (127 cm)
D = 8 inches (20 cm)	A = 0

FM = .84 (from table; using the criteria of 4 lifts per minute, duration of ≤ 1 hour, V ≥ 30 inches [76 cm])

CM = 1.0 (from table; using the criteria of good coupling and V ≥ 30 in [76 cm])

$$\text{RWL} = 51 \times (10/30) \times [1 - (.0075\ |50 - 30|)] \times [.82 + (1.8/8)] \times 1 \times .84 \times 1$$

$$= 51 \times .33 \times .85 \times 1.045 \times .84$$

$$= 12.56 \text{ pounds } (5.7 \text{ kg})$$

Discussion

The actual weight of the object being lifted is 2.3 kg (5 pounds), well below the 5.4-kg (12-pound) AL calculated by the 1981 formula and the 5.7-kg (12.56-pound) RWL calculated by the 1991 formula. Clearly there are more risk factors for Harold in performing this job than lifting the food tray. For someone with Harold's diagnosis, activities that involve repetitive forward flexion should be avoided. This example demonstrates an important concept for evaluators of work sites. The NIOSH formula was designed to be used as a guideline only and is not the only factor to be considered in the evaluation of a workstation. The lifting formula does, however, provide a work-site evaluator with a way to break the lifting task into components. Analysis of the task variables of both calculations shows that the horizontal multiplier causes the greatest reduction in each LC (.2 in the 1981 formula and .33 in the 1991 formula). Figure 8–6 shows that the horizontal reach of the job is of greatest concern.

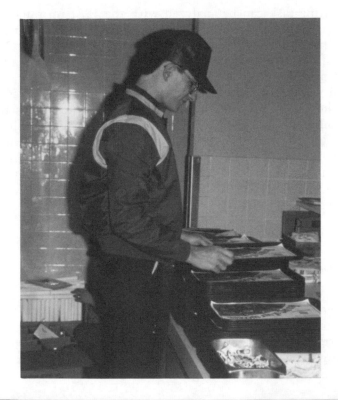

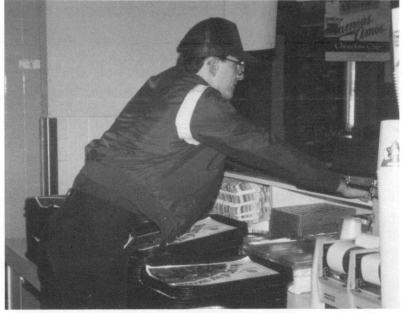

Figure 8–6   Fast-food worker handing food tray to customer.

This lifting task can be analyzed with the 1981 formula because no asymmetric twisting is involved in the lift. When the 1991 formula is used, the asymmetric and coupling multipliers are not a factor ($A = 0$; $CM = 1$). For this job, the difference between the 1981 AL (12 pounds [5.4 kg]) and the 1991 RWL (12.56 pounds [5.7 kg]) is negligible.

Harold was never successful in returning to work as a fast-food employee. He did benefit from education in proper body mechanics and learned how to stabilize his back when performing the tray-lifting job. However, Harold could not tolerate the constant standing and repetitive movements involved in all aspects of fast-food work. He moved from a cold to a warm climate and assumed a job as a bookstore manager. He reported that he finds the warm climate better for his back than the cold climate.

Case Study 2

Job Description

Bob is a 32-year-old worker at a large medical center. His job in the linen service department was evaluated after he sustained a work-related back injury. The most essential job task requires him to load bags of wet laundry from the bottom of several laundry chutes to a linen cart. The revised NIOSH lifting formula was selected during the task analysis because asymmetric lifting was observed on the job (Figure 8–7).

Job Analysis

FM = .13 (from table; frequency = 10 lifts per minute; duration = 6

H origin = 20 inches (51 cm)	V origin = 18 inches (46 cm)
H destination = 20 inches (51 cm)	V destination = 52 inches (132 cm)
D = 34 inches (86 cm)	A = 50 degrees

hours/day)

CM = 1.0 (good coupling)

Actual weight of the linen bags = 30 pounds (13.6 kg)

$$RWL(org) = 51 \times (10 / H) \times [1 - (.0075 |V - 30|)] \times [.82 + (1.8 / D)] \times (1 - .0032A) \times FM \times CM$$

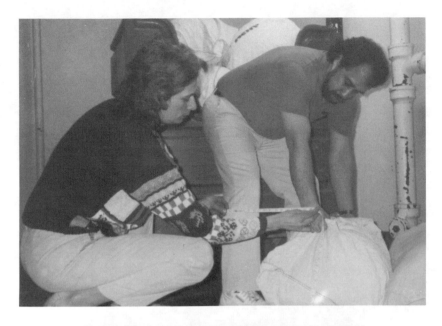

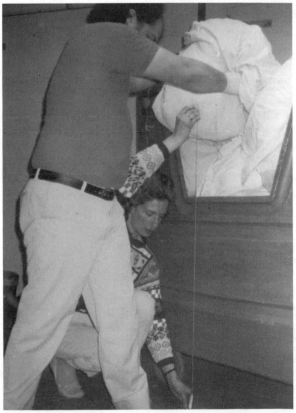

Figure 8–7   Hospital laundry worker performing asymmetric lift.

$$= 51 \times (10 / 20) \times [1 - (.0075 |18 - 30|)] \times [.82 + (1.8 / 34)] \times \{1 - [.0032 (0)]\} \\ \times .13 \times 1$$

$$= 51 \times .5 \times .91 \times .87 \times 1 \times .13 \times 1$$

$$= 2.6 \text{ pounds } (1.2 \text{ kg})$$

$$\text{RWL(dest)} = 51 \times (10 / H) \times [1 - (.0075 |V - 30|)] \times [.82 + (1.8 / D)] \\ \times (1 - .0032A) \times FM \times CM$$

$$= 51 \times (10 / 20) \times [1 - (.0075 |52 - 30|)] \times [.82 + (1.8/34)] \\ \times \{1 - [.0032 (50)]\} \times .13 \times 1$$

$$= 51 \times .5 \times .84 \times .87 \times .84 \times .13$$

$$= 2 \text{ pounds } (0.9 \text{ kg})$$

$$\text{LI (origin)} = L / RWL = 30/2.6 = 11.5$$

$$\text{LI (destination)} = L / RWL = 30/2 = 15$$

Discussion

The LI reveals the high-risk nature of performing repetitive lifting jobs. In this case, the worker lifts 12 to 15 times the RWL. In the analysis of the task variables, the factor that reduces the LC the most is the frequency multiplier (.13). Adding another worker to help perform this job in addition to slowing the frequency of lifting would raise the frequency multiplier and allow overworked muscles a chance to rest between repetitive lifts. The horizontal factor of .5 reduces the LC and could be increased by asking the workers to hold the linen bags closer to the body. The workers are reluctant to do so because the bags are wet and sometimes bloody. Providing full-cover body aprons would provide the protection necessary and encourage the workers to hug the soft linen bags to the body. The asymmetry variable could be eliminated with education in proper body mechanics—twisting is not essential to perform the job.

Conclusion

Therapists who perform work-site evaluations find that the revised NIOSH lifting formula has greater applicability to industrial work settings than its predecessor. However, because the formula is a guideline only and typically describes only one part of a worker's job, therapists should be conservative in the degree of importance they place on the formula's results. The NIOSH lifting formula is an objective evaluation tool that should be combined with careful observation of the worker's postures and positions when performing the job. In addition, NIOSH warns that the revised lifting formula needs to be validated through research before it is assumed that implementation of the formula's guidelines will reduce the risk of injuries to the lower part of the back (Waters et al, 1993). Therapists are encouraged to use the formula when working with industry to help facilitate the research process.

References

Accident Facts (1988). Chicago: National Safety Council.

Ayoub, M.M. (1991). Psychophysical basis for manual lifting guidelines. In Scientific Support Documentation for the Revised 1991 NIOSH Lifting Equation: Technical Contract Reports. NIOSH Technical Report PB91-226274. Washington, D.C.: National Institute for Occupational Safety and Health.

Batti'e, M.C., Bigos, S.J., Fisher, L.D., Hansson, T.H., James, M.E., Wortley, M.D. (1989). Isometric lifting strength as a predictor of industrial back pain reports. Spine, 14:851-856.

Department of Labor Bureau of Labor and Statistics (1982). Back injuries associated with lifting. Bulletin No. 2144. Washington, D.C.: U.S. Department of Labor.

Drury, C.G., Deeb, J.M., Hartman, B., Wooley, S., Drury, C.E., Gallagher, S. (1989). Symmetric and asymmetric manual materials handling. 1. Physiology and psychophysics. Ergonomics, 32:467-489.

Garg, A. (1989). An evaluation of the NIOSH guidelines for manual lifting with specific reference to horizontal distance. American Industrial Hygiene Association Journal, 50:157-164.

Garg, A. (1991a). Biomechanical Basis for Manual Lifting Guidelines. In Scientific Support Documentation for the Revised 1991 NIOSH Lifting Equation: Technical Contract Reports. NIOSH Technical Report PB91-226274. Washington, D.C.: National Institute for Occupational Safety and Health.

Garg, A. (1991b). Epidemiological Basis for Manual Lifting Guidelines. In Scientific Support Documentation for the Revised 1991 NIOSH Lifting Equation: Technical Contract Reports. NIOSH Technical Report PB91-226274. Washington, D.C.: National Institute for Occupational Safety and Health.

Garg, A., Badger, D. (1986). Maximum acceptable weights and maximum voluntary strength for asymmetric lifting. Ergonomics, 29:879-892.

Garg, A., Banaag, J. (1988). Maximum acceptable weights, heart rates, and RPEs for one hour's repetitive asymmetric lifting. Ergonomics, 31:77-96.

Garg, A., Chaffin, D.B., Herrin, G.D. (1978). Prediction of metabolic rates for manual materials handling jobs. American Industrial Hygiene Journal, 39:661-674.

Garg, A., Hagglund, G., Mericle, K. (1983). Physical fatigue and stresses in warehouse operations. U.S. Department of Health and Human Services, NIOSH Contract No. 210-81-6008, Technical Report. Cincinnati: National Institute for Occupational Safety and Health.

Garg, A., Saxena, U. (1980). Container characteristics and maximum acceptable weight of lift. Human Factors, 22:487-495.

Liles, D.H., Mahajan, P. (1985). Using NIOSH lifting guide decreases risks of back injuries. Occupational Health and Safety, (February) 57-60.

Mitral, A., Fard, H.F. (1986). Psychophysical and physiological responses to lifting symmetrically and asymmetrically. Ergonomics, 29:1263-1272.

National Institute for Occupational Safety and Health (1981). Work practices guide for manual lifting. U.S. Department of Health and Human Services, NIOSH Technical Report No. 81-122. Cincinnati: National Institute for Occupational Safety and Health.

National Institute for Occupational Safety and Health (1986). Proposed National Strategy for the Prevention of Musculoskeletal Injuries. U.S. Department of Health and Human Services. Cincinnati: National Institute of Occupational Safety and Health.

Punnett, L., Fine, L.J., Keyserling, W.M., Herrin, G.D., Chaffin, D.B. (1987). A Case-referent Study of Back Disorders in Automobile Assembly Workers: The Health Effects of Nonneutral Trunk Postures. Ann Arbor: University of Michigan Center for Ergonomics.

Putz-Anderson, V., Waters, T.R. (1991). Revisions in the NIOSH guide to manual lifting. Presented at the National Conference for a National Strategy for Occupational Musculoskeletal Injury Prevention: Implementation Issues and Research Needs, Ann Arbor, April 1991.

Rodgers, S.H., Yates, J.W. (1991). Physiological basis for manual lifting guidelines. In Scientific Support Documentation for the Revised 1991 NIOSH Lifting Equation: Technical Contract Reports. NIOSH Technical Report PB91-226274. Washington, D.C.: National Institute for Occupational Safety and Health.

Ruhman, H., Schmidtke, H. (1989). Human strength: Measurements of maximum isometric forces in industry. Ergonomics, 32:865-879.

Smith, J.L., Jiang, B.C. (1984). A manual materials handling study of bag lifting. American Industrial Hygiene Association Journal, 45:505-508.

Snook, S.H., Ciriello, V.M. (1991). The design of manual handling tasks: Revised tables. Ergonomics, 34:1197-1213.

Waters, T.R., Putz-Anderson, V., Garg, A., Fine, L. (1993). Revised NIOSH equation for the design and evaluation of manual lifting tasks. Ergonomics, 36:749-776.

CHAPTER 9

Seating

Diane C. Hermenau

ABSTRACT

Because of the proliferation of computers in offices and factories, jobs are evolving from multidimensional to unidimensional, causing workers to sit for long periods of time. Consequently, seating has become a critical aspect of the workplace. A poorly designed computer workstation puts workers at risk for back, neck, shoulder, forearm, wrist, hand, and leg injuries. Therapists with expertise in seating have found this to be an area in which consultation is frequently required. Research reveals that disk pressures are greater when a person is sitting than when he or she is standing. Radiographic studies show that the pelvis rotates backward and the lumbar spine flattens in sitting. Electromyographic studies support the finding that sitting in a slouched or reclining position relaxes the trunk muscles and requires minimal muscle activity to hold the body weight in balance. However, disk pressures are greatest when a person sits in a slouched posture. Therefore, prolonged sitting in poor posture puts workers at risk for injuries. Good ergonomic chair design features easily adjustable seat height and backrest and seat support and inclination to correct posture and provide comfort for worker health and safety. High backrests, armrests, and footrests are optional features, the need for which must be determined after the tasks are analyzed to ensure compatibility between the chair selected and the tasks performed. A wide variety of seating options exist, including the saddle seat, kneeling chair, sit-stand workstations, and use of devices such as lumbar supports, wedges, and back slings. All of these seating options are focused on the goal of promoting correct posture and worker comfort while increasing productivity and reducing injuries

---

Ergonomics is the art and science of fitting the worker to the work, of facilitating the worker-machine interface. With the proliferation in the use of personal computers, this relationship between work and worker is achieving increased importance as more workers sit in front of terminals to do their work. Therapists are in a pivotal place to assist industry in designing optimal workstations for workers, which now more than ever involves seating.

About three-fourths of all workers in industrialized countries have sedentary jobs (Grandjean, 1988). Sedentary work is defined by the *Dictionary of Occupational Titles*, published by the United States Department of Labor, as "exerting up to 10 pounds of force occasionally and/or a negligible amount of force frequently or constantly to lift, carry, push and pull, or otherwise move objects, including the human body. Sedentary work involves sitting most of the time, but may involve walking or standing for brief periods of time. Jobs are sedentary if walking and standing are required only occasionally and all other sedentary criteria are met" (United States Department of Labor, 1991, p. 1013). Seated tasks require or feature the following characteristics: visual acuity; repetitive movements, particularly fine manipulation of the forearms and hands; and sitting for more than 4 hours (Eastman Kodak, 1983).

Jobs that once had a wide variety of tasks, which allowed workers to get up from their work areas and change body positions, now require sitting for long periods. This sharp contrast is apparent in industries such as banking, insurance, publishing, and airlines. Computers are now being used by clerical workers, dispatchers, machine operators, medical workers, and in numerous other situations. Consequently, workers are spending more and more time in fixed postures in front of computer terminals. Thus, the chair they use takes on great importance.

This chapter discusses the biomechanics of sitting, the risks related to prolonged sitting and poor posture, the features of ergonomic chair design, how to fit worker and workstation together, indications for seated work, and special considerations, including use of a video display terminal (VDT), the sit-stand position, kneeling chairs, and lumbar supports. The focus is on office and industrial seating.

Considerations of Sitting

Researchers began studying the effects of the seated position in the 1940s. Sitting has been defined as a position in which the weight of the body is transferred to a supporting area, mainly by the ischial tuberosities of the pelvis and their surrounding soft tissues (Schoberth, 1962). In sitting, most of the body weight is on the seat, back, and feet.

A brief review of anatomy is helpful to fully appreciate the biomechanics of sitting. Thirty-three vertebrae compose the spine. They are the cervical, thoracic, and lumbar vertebrae, the sacrum, and the coccyx. In standing, the spine forms three natural curves: the cervical curve is inward (lordosis); the thoracic curve is outward (kyphosis); and the lumbar curve is inward (lordosis). The cervical and lumbar portions of the spine are mobile in relation to the thoracic spine. The intervertebral disks are located between the vertebrae. They act as shock absorbers between the vertebrae and provide flexibility to the spine. A disk is made up of viscous fluid contained by a tough, fibrous outside wall. Ligaments provide stability to the vertebrae and are located on the anterior and posterior walls of the spine. Muscles along the spine maintain posture and provide stability to the trunk. The nerves that compose the spinal cord are protected by the vertebrae and pass to the extremities, allowing motor and sensory information to pass to and from the brain. Blood flows along the spine, but the blood supply to the disks is limited.

The sacrum is essentially fixed and moves in relation to the pelvis; therefore, pelvic movement affects the shape of the lumbar spine. A forward or anterior rotation of the pelvis causes the lumbar spine to move toward increased lordosis to maintain an upright trunk. When the pelvis is tilted backward, the lumbar spine tends to flatten, sometimes causing kyphosis. Radiographic studies have verified that the pelvis rotates backward and the lumbar spine flattens during sitting (Åkerblom, 1948; Burandt, 1969; Carlsoo, 1972; Keegan, 1953; Schoberth, 1962; Umezawa, 1971; Rosemeyer, 1972; Andersson et al, 1979). Disk pressures also change dramatically when a person moves from standing to sitting upright to sitting slouched. Nachemson and Elfstrom (1970) and Andersson and Ortengren (1974) developed methods to measure disk pressure. They found that disk pressure is greater during sitting than during standing. Nachemson and Morris (1964) published data on in vivo disk pressure measurements of people who stood and sat without support. The pressures measured when the subjects were standing were found to be about 35% lower than those when the subjects were sitting. Research also demonstrates that increased disk pressure means that the disks are being overloaded and will wear out more quickly (Grandjean, 1988).

Disk pressures drop with inclination of the backrest of a chair, especially when the backrest is tilted from vertical to 110 degrees (Andersson & Ortengren, 1974). The backrest inclination is defined as the angle between the seat and the backrest. Through research it has been found that disk pressures are lower when a person is sitting and leaning back 110 to 120 degrees and using a 50-mm lumbar pad than when standing in normal lumbar lordosis (Andersson & Ortengren, 1974).

Muscle activity has been extensively researched through electromyography (EMG) of the back muscles during standing and sitting. Studies by Lundervold (1951 a,b; 1958) and Floyd and Roberts (1958) found that the myoelectric activity was less when the back support was located in the lumbar region rather than in the thoracic region. This confirmed a finding by Åkerblom (1948) that a support in the lumbar region is as effective as a full back support. Research has provided a dichotomy: disk pressures are reduced when a person sits in erect posture and maintains the three natural spinal curves, but the trunk muscles exert less energy when a person sits in a slightly flexed or slouched position.

Zacharokow (1988) has done extensive research to support the theory that it is necessary to support the sacrum and the lower thoracic spine to achieve proper sitting posture. The rationale behind sacral–lower thoracic support when sitting is that the proper axial relation between the thorax and the pelvis must be restored by bringing the upper trunk over the hips.

Zacharokow pointed out that sitting is a dynamic activity. People sit on their ischial tuberosities, and this causes the pelvis to rock. Without sacral support to produce an anterior tilt to the pelvis, the sacrum rotates posteriorly, bringing the lumbar spine into a flattened or kyphotic position. Zacharokow suggested that the use of a lumbar support with a seat backrest inclination of 110 to 120 degrees causes the worker doing close work to be too far from the surface. This requires flexion of the neck and upper body to compensate, increasing stress to these areas. Many therapists agree. Zacharokow designed a seating system, the Zack Back Posture Chair, to alleviate this problem.

A lumbar support may not be effective when the task is writing or close work at a table top or bench. A study by Steward and McQuilton (1987) found that a position of balanced pelvic muscle groups allows the body to be positioned over the ischial tuberosities (as in horseback riding) and not behind the seat base. This balance promotes greater accuracy in hand function and preservation of the lumbar curve.

Cervical Spine and Shoulders

The line of vision dictates head and neck posture. If the work surface is too low, or the computer screen is too far away from the user, the result is neck and trunk flexion. If the head is held forward, increased cervical muscle activity is needed to support the weight of the head and results in increased muscle fatigue. Because of the increased use of computers, more workers are complaining of neck and shoulder pain. The complaints are becoming as common as complaints of low-back pain. Diagnoses related to such injuries include shoulder and neck muscle strain, degenerative disk disease, and overuse syndrome. In Japan, these conditions are considered occupational diseases because they are often seen in typists, telephone and cash register operators, and assembly-plant workers (Grandjean, 1988).

Studies of VDT operators reveal that although the small muscles of the forearms and hands undergo almost constant dynamic contractions, the proximal muscles of the shoulders and neck provide postural support through static contraction. Prolonged static muscle contraction can cause considerable fatigue. Onishi et al (1982) studied the EMG activity of the trapezius muscle during keyboard operations and found that when activity was present, the static loading of the trapezius muscle reached 20 to 30% of the level of maximum contraction.

Because the keyboard is the primary piece of equipment involved in the worker-machine interface, the correct relationship is of prime importance. Keyboard height is directly related to static loading of the trapezius muscle. Shoulder strain in keyboard workers is also related to forearm angle. Erdelyi et al (1988) found a reduction in the static load of the trapezius muscle when the forearms were at an angle of at least 100 degrees. A properly adjusted armrest can provide the arm support necessary to reduce the level of myoelectric activity in the neck and shoulder muscles. Andersson et al (1974) found that the myoelectric activity was reduced in the lumbar region and the cervical and thoracic regions with a backrest inclination of 110 to 120 degrees.

Proper work surface height is important. If the work surface is too high, elbow flexion and shoulder abduction and elevation occur. This puts stress on the shoulder joints and increases the fatigue of the neck and shoulder muscles. The recommended position for desk work is shoulder abduction of 15 to 20 degrees or less and shoulder flexion of 25 degrees or less (Engdahl, 1978).

Legs

Legs increase in volume by 4% over a workday (Winkel, 1978; 1981). A chair that is too high or a seat pan that is too deep places pressure on the thighs and the back of the knees and can cause compression of the sciatic nerve. This increases the tendency toward swelling in the legs, ankles, and feet. A chair that is too high causes the worker to lean forward to support the feet on the floor. Consequently, the back of the chair is not used, and the individual sits in an unsupported position. A chair that is too low causes the hips and knees to flex beyond 90 degrees. This results in a posterior pelvic tilt and lumbar flattening as well as a decrease in diaphragmatic breathing, which leads to low energy.

The best way to avoid problems is to adjust the seat height so that the feet rest firmly on the floor or on a footrest. There should be 2.5 cm (1 inch) of space between the seat edge and the back of the knees. A worker can avoid swelling in the feet by taking frequent breaks; movement every 15 minutes can reduce swelling up to 2.3% (Winkel, 1978; 1981).

Ergonomics of Sitting

People who sit for prolonged periods are at risk for back injury for the following reasons:

1. Strained ligaments and stretching of muscles over time cause low-back pain
2. About 60% of adults have a backache at least once in their lives, and the most common cause is disk trouble (Grandjean, 1988)
3. Flattening of the lumbar spine during sitting causes disk herniation

It is important for therapists to emphasize to managers in industry that although workers reduce the static muscular activity required on their hips, knees, ankles, and feet when sitting as opposed to standing, they put more strain on their backs, especially the lower part, when sitting. When working in industry, therapists should promote the use of correct sitting posture and emphasize the following health benefits of good posture:

1. A decrease in ligamentous strain to prevent overstretching
2. A decrease in muscular strain and overstretching of the back muscles, which causes muscle imbalances
3. A decrease in intradiskal pressure
4. A healthy spine along the whole kinetic chain because of a reduction in stress on the thoracic and cervical spine and shoulder girdle
5. More efficient muscle work and a reduction in fatigue because muscles are at a mechanical advantage because the postural muscles are used to support the spine and rib cage while the extremities are used to conduct work
6. A greater range of motion of the upper extremities when the worker reaches to shoulder level and overhead because the upper body is not flexed, which limits this range
7. Efficient diaphragmatic breathing because there is a greater distance between the sternum and pelvis
8. More air entering the lungs because breathing increases, providing more oxygenated blood to vital organs, including the brain. Efficient breathing diminishes fatigue, resulting in increased productivity and accurate work

9. Improved lower-extremity circulation with proper seat tilt and depth
10. Good posture, which promotes a positive self-image

It is important for therapists to have a thorough understanding of the biomechanics of sitting, so that they can assist industrial managers with workstation design. Therapists must be keenly aware of the type of tasks being performed by the worker. For example, writing at a desk and keying into a computer may require different seating solutions. It is also important to keep in mind the broad variations in workers' body sizes and dimensions and individual personal sitting habits and movement patterns. Each of these factors influences the selection of the chair and other equipment.

The components of most office or industrial chairs are as follows:

1. Seat (width and depth)
2. Backrest
3. Pedestal base (seat height)
4. Four- or five-prong base with or without casters
5. Tension adjustment for forward and backward inclination of tilted backrest
6. Armrests and a foot ring (optional)

Common Problems with the Typical Office or Industrial Chair

1. The backrest is not easily adjustable and offers limited range of adjustment to provide adequate support to the lower part of the back. Often, the industrial chair is not padded; consequently sharp edges come in contact with the user.
2. The seat height adjustment is controlled by spinning the seat clockwise to raise it or counterclockwise to lower it. The worker must be out of the chair to do this.
3. The tension control knob is often difficult to reach because it is under or behind the seat. Most workers are unfamiliar with the purpose of this tension control knob, and therefore it is rarely used.
4. If the chair has armrests, they are often too wide, too low, or too high to be used while the worker is at a work surface. If the armrests are too high, they interfere with the ability to pull the chair under the work surface. This forces the worker to sit forward on the seat. Consequently, the backrest is not used, and the worker sits unsupported.
5. The seat may be too deep for short people; the consequence is that their feet dangle and their backs are unsupported.

Good Ergonomic Chair Design

In the selection of an ergonomically appropriate chair, the most important feature is adjustability. The adjustments must be easy to make and the controls must be accessible to the worker while he or she is seated in the chair. The purchaser must be aware that some manufacturers advertise a chair as "ergonomic" simply because it has pneumatic seat-height adjustment. These chairs may not meet the other criteria for an ergonomically correct chair. Even if a chair is labeled ergonomic and meets the American National Standards Institute/Human Factors Society (ANSI/HFS) standards, it may not be comfortable for all workers. The standards are minimal and do not apply to 10% of the population because the standards pertain to the 5th to the 95th (smallest to largest) percentile of the population according to anthropometric data. Therefore, a company that wants to maintain uniformity should select a chair that comes in more than one size.

A number of recommendations have been published with regard to anthropometric data related to seating design, that is, dimensions, backrest, and seat-height adjustability (Chaffin & Andersson, 1984; Eastman Kodak, 1983, 1986). The data differ from country to country because of the physical dimensions of individuals within a population.

Dynamic is a term used to describe an ergonomic chair. It indicates that the chair is capable of leaning forward and backward and that the backrest inclination can be easily adjusted. Beyond this requirement chairs differ widely. Some feature a "dynamic" forward tilt of the seat pan and backrest inclination as a unit; others feature an adjustable backrest inclination with seat tilt; still others feature a backrest and seat that adjust independently of each other. Some chairs allow the user to lock into a preferred position by means of static posture settings. Other chairs have a free-flowing (dynamic-motion) design and continuously move with the user. Consideration must be given to the nature of the tasks done while sitting and the personal habits and preferences of the user.

People sit in different postures to perform different tasks. Therefore, an ergonomic chair fits comfortably while the worker performs various tasks and is not locked into one position.

In the budgets of most companies, chairs are capital equipment. An ergonomically correct office or industrial chair can cost as much $1200. However, a good chair with pneumatic seat-height adjustment, an adjustable backrest, and a tilting seat pan costs about $250. Costs increase depending on the number of adjustable features and the fabric selected. It is advisable for the therapist to have various office or industrial chairs available in the clinic or workplace for workers to try. People need time to get used to different chairs that promote correct posture, especially if they have been sitting in poor posture for a long time.

The therapist can influence industry by educating managers, supervisors, purchasing agents, and employees about what to look for when evaluating and selecting new chairs. Therapists should encourage employers to involve their employees in the evaluation and selection process. The features of an ergonomically well-designed chair are as follows:

1. The seat height is easily adjustable, as in a pneumatic chair
2. The backrest is easily adjustable to support the lumbar spine vertically (height) and horizontally (forward and backward) and is narrow enough so that the operator's arms or torso do not strike it if rotation is required
3. The seat tilts forward and backward independently of the backrest. This feature is useful with fine detail work and office work
4. The seat edge is curved to reduce pressure under the legs
5. There is enough space between the back of the chair and the seat to accommodate the buttocks
6. The adjustable armrests (optional) are small and low enough to fit under the work surface and to support the back when the worker works close to the work surface
7. The base has five points (for safety)
8. The worker can make adjustments easily with one hand while seated
9. The upholstery fabric is comfortable, reduces heat transfer in warm climates and static electricity in cold weather, and is stain resistant or easily cleaned
10. Training is provided to ensure that workers are familiar with the features and adjustments of an optimally fitting chair.

A chair assessment is helpful to allow employers and employees to evaluate various chairs. An example of one such assessment is in Appendix 9–1. The guidelines for an ergonomically well-designed chair are specified in Figure 9–1.

An ergonomically correct chair, like all ergonomic equipment, will not be used if the worker does not know how to use it well. Workers must be trained in the proper use of the chair or workstation so that they are knowledgeable about the capabilities of the equipment. An excellent role for therapists who consult in industry is to help educate purchasing agents, managers, and chief executive officers on the medical cost savings of purchasing adjustable equipment and then teaching employees how to use it.

Work Height

Frequently an employer asks how high a desk, table, or countertop should be. This question is critical when an employer is designing new workstations. Information regarding recommended work surface heights has been provided by Eastman Kodak (1983). In many situations, the workstation is fixed; for example, desks are permanent or countertops and shelves are built-in. In these situations, the chair is the most flexible and usually the most critical piece of equipment to adjust or change for a better worker-to-workstation fit.

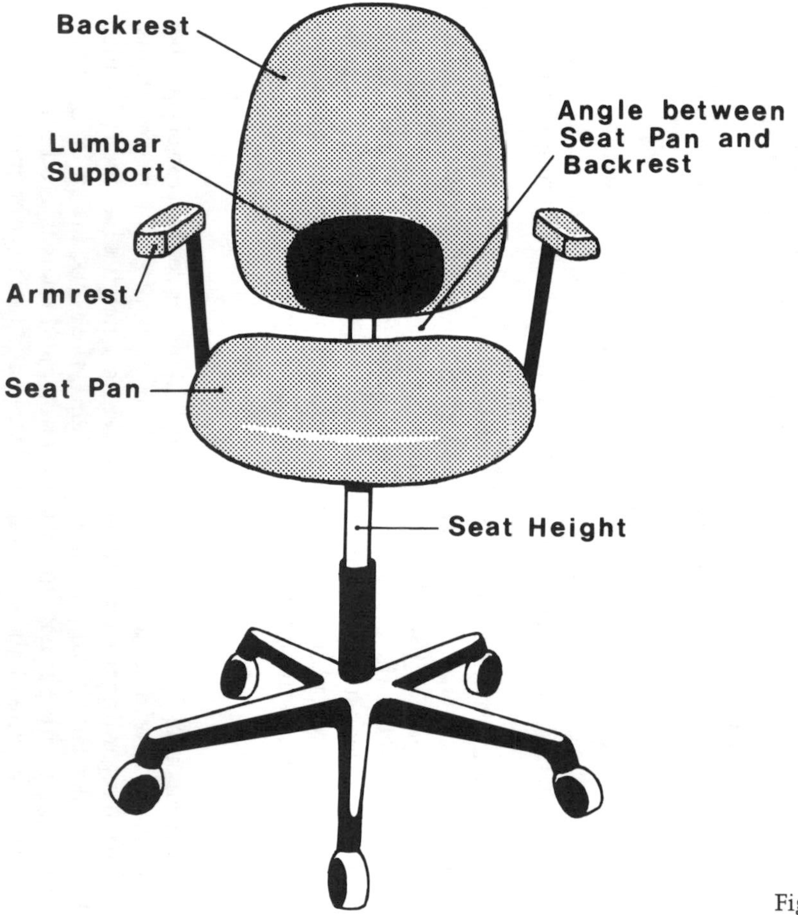

ERGONOMIC DESIGN GUIDELINES

Seat Pan	
height	15" - 22" (range of adjustability)
width	17" - 19"
depth	minimum 17"
slope	0-7° (range of adjustability)
contour	waterfall front
Backrest	
height	6" - 20"
width	13" - 14"
lumbar support	4" - 10" *
up/down	7" - 10" *
in/out (forward)	12" - 17"*
tilt angle	5 - 30°
Seat pan/back	90 - 105°
Armrest	
height	7" - 11" *
length	6" - 10"
width	2" minimum
Support, swivel	five star base
Material and padding	permeable

* measured relative to chair seat

Backrest

Angle between Seat Pan and Backrest

Lumbar Support

Armrest

Seat Pan

Seat Height

Figure 9–1   Ergonomic design guidelines for a chair.

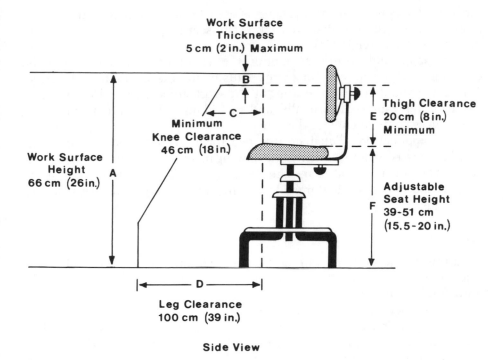

Work Surface
Thickness
5 cm (2 in.) Maximum

B

C

Minimum
Knee Clearance
46 cm (18 in.)

Work Surface
Height
66 cm (26 in.)   A

Thigh Clearance
E 20 cm (8 in.)
Minimum

Adjustable
Seat Height
F 39-51 cm
(15.5-20 in.)

D

Leg Clearance
100 cm (39 in.)

Side View

Figure 9–2 Recommended dimensions for a seated workplace without a footrest. (Reprinted courtesy of Eastman Kodak Company.)

The working height depends on the nature of the tasks performed. Tasks such as writing or light assembly are most easily performed if the work is at elbow height. If the job requires fine detail and visual acuity, it may be necessary to raise the work to bring it closer to the eyes (Eastman Kodak, 1983).

After a worker and workstation have been fit to each other, consideration must be given to the layout of items frequently used. Items at the workstation should be within a comfortable reaching distance. A good rule is to place items within an arm's length or within the radius of both arms. Therefore, frequently used items, such as a telephone, dictation equipment, computer and keyboard, calculator, reference materials, or files should be situated to achieve this proximity. Removing clutter is frequently recommended by installing overhead shelving, storage shelving, or additional file cabinets

Armrests

Armrests are recommended for assembly or repair tasks when the arm has to be held away from the body and is not moved extensively during the work cycle (Eastman Kodak, 1983). EMG studies substantiate lowered trapezius muscle activity when armrest support is used. Disk pressure is reduced when armrests are used, provided the backrest-to-seat angle is not too large (Andersson & Ortengren, 1974).

Nonadjustable armrests are often too wide for the average person and too high for a person with long arms, causing increased shoulder elevation. Armrests should be near the front of the worksurface, should tilt without having to be readjusted manually, and should be cushioned to avoid having sharp edges come in contact the skin.

An application of chairs with specialized armrests is evident in the textile industry, where workers sit at sewing machines for prolonged periods. Some VDT operators also are choosing to use elbow or forearm rests to support the upper arm and provide free movement of the forearms, wrists, and hands.

Footrests

To allow for workers of various sizes, a workstation should include an adjustable footrest. Footrests come in a variety of styles—fixed or portable, horizontal, as in a platform, or tilted. Chairs with a foot ring may not be satisfactory because the ring is often close to the floor and fixed. If a short person were to raise the chair, he or she would be unable to reach the foot ring. Some chairs are manufactured with foot rings that move with the seat as it is adjusted, and others have foot rings that can be adjusted independently. Portable footrests must be large enough to support the soles of both feet. A surface of 30 × 41 cm (12 × 16 inches) with an angle of 25 to 30 degrees and a nonskid surface is recommended (Roebuck et al, 1975). If the footrest is built into the workplace, it should be 30 cm (12 inches) deep and wide enough to reach across the width of the seat. Built-in footrests in a workplace where the board can be varied in 5-cm (2-inch) increments (like a bookshelf) are recommended (Eastman Kodak, 1983).

A variety of footrests are available and may be found in many office and industrial supply catalogues. Telephone books are an inexpensive solution, or footrests can be built inexpensively from wood scraps. Workers often say footrests help remind them to sit up straighter. This is the tactile reminder to use better posture, regardless of the chair.

Special Considerations: Workstation Design for Seated Workers

Workers Who Use Video Display Terminals

Poorly designed VDT workstations put workers at risk for not only back injuries but also neck, shoulder, forearm, wrist and hand, and leg problems. Visual problems are also becoming widely reported. With the proliferation of VDTs, office work has been transformed. The most common obstacle confronting an employer in dealing with this office transformation is the new

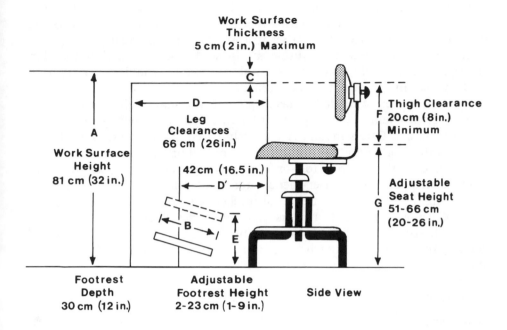

Figure 9–3   Recommended dimensions for a seated workplace with a footrest. (Reprinted courtesy of Eastman Kodak Company.)

technology. The computer is phased in as the old machinery (typewriter) is phased out. During an office work-site evaluation the therapist often finds an L-shaped desk with a drop for an electric typewriter, a telephone, a calculator, desk references, ledgers, or files. The worker's chair is typically a "steno" chair, which features a small backrest with limited adjustability. After the new equipment arrives, this same workstation must house a computer terminal, hard drive, printer, and keyboard, which range in size and adjustability. Older-model computers are larger and limited in adjustability. The introduction of the computer not only necessitates prolonged sitting but also has produced a cramped workspace, because a computer occupies a great deal of desktop space. In addition, the drop that is a good height for a typewriter is typically too low for a computer terminal and keyboard.

Hunting and Grandjean (1976) conducted a study of office chairs. They compared three chairs: a tiltable chair with a high backrest, a similar model with a fixed seat, and a traditional chair with an adjustable but short backrest. The survey indicated that after using each of the three chairs for 2 weeks, office workers preferred the two chairs with a high backrest. A high backrest allows the user to lean back and supports the body weight. It was also noted that the tilting feature was not desirable in that most users wanted a fixed position once they found a position of comfort. This research supports the findings of studies discussed earlier in this chapter, which suggest reduced disk pressure and reduced muscle strain with backrest inclination. For example, when driving a car for several hours, one would rather sit back slightly than in an upright trunk posture.

The ergonomic chair has been become the main solution for office workplace problems. A poorly fitting chair affects all other aspects of the worker-to-workstation match. A correctly fitted chair affects the relation between the worker and the workstation, and all other components should be evaluated when the chair-to-worker fit is completed. Employers may want to invest in better-quality user-friendly adjustable chairs as a first step toward improving the workplace, since most budgets are not generous to the point of purchasing equipment such as ergonomic desks or computer stands. However, studies confirm that worktables with an adjustable height and desktop inclination, along with ergonomic chairs, increase worker comfort and, as a consequence, productivity.

Finding the Fit Between Worker and Workstation

When determining the fit between a worker and a VDT workstation, the best and easiest method to teach is a kinesthetic or tactile approach, wherein workers feel their body in relation to the machine (computer, keyboard, and terminal). The worker assumes the correct sitting posture: hip, knee, and ankle joints flexed to 90 degrees; feet firmly on floor; shoulder girdle over hip girdle; and head over shoulders to achieve the three natural spinal curves. The worker then adjusts the backrest for proper lumbar support or uses a lumbar cushion, towel roll, or seat wedge to achieve proper lumbosacral support. The distance from the worker to the screen dictates head position. The ergonomic literature suggests a viewing distance of 51 to 76 cm (20 to 30 inches) (Pinsky, 1987). An arm's reach is an easy reference point.

Arm rests or wrist rests are recommended to decrease shoulder muscle fatigue. A document holder attached to the screen allows lateral eye gaze as opposed to repetitive neck flexion and extension to look at work on a desktop surface. A footrest may be used either to support the feet of a short worker or to change leg position during prolonged sitting. Shoulders should be relaxed, flexed 25 degrees or less, and abducted 20 to 25 degrees or less. Elbows are held comfortably by the sides and flexed to 90 to 100 degrees. Forearms and wrists are in a neutral position, and the fingers and thumbs are comfortably flexed.

Lighting, climate control, ventilation, workspace layout and storage, work breaks, and employee health and safety for VDT operators are other important considerations in the analysis of a modern office (see chapter 5).

A variety of educational sessions are presented to workers to achieve worker compliance and follow-through. These sessions typically include a brief spinal anatomy lesson (including a discussion of disk pressure); the importance of proper sitting posture; the correct use of body mechanics while sitting, such as the avoidance of bending and twisting; and mechanisms of injury to the back, neck, shoulders, wrists, hands, and legs. The therapist must be concerned with the work flow and work methods of the worker as well as individual habits, because these factors influence equipment recommendations. For example, if a worker uses a computer to access information, transfers the information into ledgers by hand, and uses a calculator intermittently, the chair requirements may be very different from those of a data processor who performs continuous keyboard work. The first worker may not need armrests or wristrests at the workstation, and the second may benefit from one or both. In addition, what is good for one worker may not be good for all. People come in all shapes and sizes. Employers serve their employees best by providing options in chair selection and in the use and selection of adaptive equipment such as headsets, elbow supports, armrests, incline boards, split keyboards, wristrests, footrests, antiglare screens, and screen hoods.

Sit-Stand Position

Sit-stand workstations should be considered when the worker must repetitively reach forward more than 41 cm (16 inches) or reach up more than 15 cm (6 inches) (Eastman Kodak, 1983). A very high chair with a forward-sloping seat can be used for a semisitting posture. This posture provides some torso support with some lumbar lordosis for work that requires mobility and reach. Most of the weight is on the buttocks and the feet when the worker uses this kind of chair. Jobs such as graphic design and drafting, which require large work surfaces, are best suited for sit-stand workstations.

Computer work has traditionally been done while sitting. However, given the long hours spent by some workers in front of a computer terminal and the wider acceptance of ergonomics in the office workplace, sit-stand computer workstations are becoming more common. Simply by pushing a button or switch, a worker can change from a sitting to a standing position. Of course, such adjustability is expensive. One such product costs $2,500; the manufacturer advertises that it accommodates user sizes from a 5th-percentile woman seated to a 95th-percentile man standing.

Kneeling Chairs

The Balans chair from Norway is probably the most famous of the half-sitting, half-kneeling posture chairs. It features a forward tilted seat and a knee support. This design results in a wider hip angle and maintains the three natural curves of the spine, thus preserving lumbar lordosis. Studies by Krueger (1984), however, found that the load on the knees and lower legs is too great and sitting becomes painful. Work surface height is also critical for proper fit. Common practice in offices that have a kneeling chair is to rotate the chair among workers, limiting each worker's use to approximately 2 hours. This system provides a change in posture for those who must sit to perform work.

Lumbar Support, Wedge, Back Sling

There are a wide variety of lumbar supports on the market. They come in the form of small, rounded, oblong pillows to full-length molded plastic frames that feature low-back and lateral support, such as the Obus chair. Most medical supply catalogues contain an array of lumbar cushions, rolls, and half-rolls. It is important for therapists to educate people in the correct support based on body type and the particular chair or seat (office, industrial, home, car) for which the cushion is intended.

The seat wedge, which comes in a variety of styles, provides the user the ischial support to tip the pelvis anteriorly when used correctly. It encourages upward posture and may be the best adaptation for a user who must sit close to a work surface to write. The seat wedge is useful in a chair that lacks a forward tilting feature and thus gives the user more variety when seated for long periods. Another simple remedy to promote an anterior pelvic tilt is to place a small towel roll under the ischial tuberosities. As the body weight is shifted forward, the upper body comes closer to the work surface, and the towel prevents the worker from rocking back on the ischial tuberosities.

A back sling is a device that works independently of the chair. Through a strapping system, which consists of a low-back cushion and slings that anchor at the knees, the lumbar spine is held in lordosis. The strapping around the knees is typically held in place with a buckle between the thighs. Consequently, female office workers are often reluctant to use it. However, this device has met with great success for workers with low-back pain who sit on industrial stools at assembly lines all day.

References

Åkerblom, B. (1948). Standing and sitting posture: With special reference to the construction of chairs. Stockholm: Nordiska Bokhandeln.

Andersson, G.B.J., Murphy, R.W., Ortengren, R., Nachemson, A.L. (1979). The influence of backrest inclination and lumbar support on the lumbar lordosis in sitting. Spine, 4:52-58.

Andersson, G.B.J., Ortengren, R. (1974). Lumbar disc pressure and myoelectric back muscle activity during sitting. 1. Studies on an experimental chair. Scandinavian Journal of Rehabilitation Medicine, 3:115-121; 104-114; 122-127; 128-135.

Burandt, U. (1969). Rontgenuntersuchung uber die Stellung von Becken und Wirbelsaule beim Sitzen auf vorgeneirten Flachen. In E. Grandjean (Ed.), Sitting Posture (pp. 242-250). London: Taylor & Francis.

Carlsoo, S. (1972). How Man Moves. Heinemann: London.

Chaffin, D., Andersson, G. (1984). Occupational Biomechanics. New York: Wiley.

Eastman Kodak (1983). Ergonomic Design for People at Work. Vol. 1. New York: Van Nostrand Reinhold.

Eastman Kodak (1986). Ergonomics Design for People at Work. Vol 2. New York: Van Nostrand Reinhold.

Engdahl, S. (1978). Specification for office furniture. In B. Jonsson (Ed.), Sitting Work Postures (pp. 97-135). No. 12. Solna, Sweden: National Board of Occupational Safety and Health, (in Swedish).

Erdelyi, A., Silhoven, T., Helin, P., et al (1988). Shoulder strain in keyboard workers and its alleviation by arm supports. International Archives of Occupational and Environmental Health, 60:119-124.

Floyd, W.F., Roberts, D.F. (1958). Anatomical and physiological principles in chair and table design. Ergonomics, 2(2):1.

Grandjean, E. (1988). Fitting the Task to the Man, 4th ed. London: Taylor & Francis.

Hunting, W., Grandjean, E. (1976). Sitzverhalten und subjektives Wohlbefinden auf schwenkbaren und fixierten Formsitzen. Zeitschrift der Arbeitswissenschaft, 30:161-164.

Keegan, J.J. (1953). Alterations of the lumbar curve related to posture and seating. Journal of Bone and Joint Surgery, 35A:589-603.

Krueger, H. (1984). Zur Ergonomie von Balans-Sitzelementen im Hinblick auf ihre Verwendbarkeit als regulare Arbeitsstuhle. Report 8092. Zurich: Department of Ergonomics, Swiss Federal Institute of Technology.

Lundervold, A.J.S. (1951a). Electromyographic investigations of position and manner of working in typewriting. Acta Orthopedica Scandinavica, Suppl. 84.

Lundervold, A.J.S. (1951b). Electromyographic investigations during sedentary work especially typewriting. British Journal of Physical Medicine, 14:31.

Lundervold, A.J.S. (1958). Electromyographic investigations during typewriting. Ergonomics, 1:226.

Nachemson, A., Elfstrom, G. (1970). Intravital dynamic pressure measurements in lumbar discs. Scandinavian Journal of Rehabilitation Medicine, Suppl. 1.

Nachemson, A., Morris, J.M. (1964). In vivo measurements of intradiscal pressure. Journal of Bone Joint Surgery, 46A:1077-1092.

Onishi, N., Sakai, K., Kogi, K. (1982). Arm and shoulder muscle load in various keyboard operating jobs of women. Journal of Human Ergology, 11:89-97.

Pinsky, M. (1987). The VDT Book: A Computer Users Guide to Health and Safety. New York: The New York Committee for Occupational Safety and Health.

Roebuck, J.A., Jr., Kroemer, K.H.E., Thomson, W.G. (1975). Engineering Anthropometry Methods. New York: Wiley.

Rosemeyer, B. (1972). Eine Methode zur Beckenfixierung im Arbeitssitz. Zeitschrift fur Orthopaedie und ihre Grenzgebiete, 110:514-517.

Schoberth, H. (1962). Sitzhaltung, Sitzschaden, Sitzmobel. Berlin: Springer.

Stewart, P., McQuilton, G. (1987). Straddle seating for the cerebral palsied child. Physiotherapy, 73:204-206.

Umezawa, F. (1971). The study of comfortable sitting postures. Journal of the Japanese Orthopedic Association, 45:1015.

United States Department of Labor (1991). Dictionary of Occupational Titles, 4th ed. Washington, D.C.: U.S.Government Printing Office.

Winkel, J. (1981). Swelling of lower leg in sedentary work: A pilot study. Journal of Human Ergology, 10:139-149.

Winkel, J. (1978). Leg problems from longlasting sitting. In B. Jonsson (Ed.), Sitting Work Postures (pp. 72-78). No. 12. Solna, Sweden: National Board of Occupational Safety and Health (in Swedish).

Zacharkow, D. (1988). Posture: Sitting, Standing, Chair Design and Exercise. Springfield, Ill.: Charles C. Thomas.

Suggested Reading

American National Standard for Human Factors Engineering of Visual Display Terminal Workstations (1988). ANSI/HFS Standard No. 100-1988. Santa Monica: The Human Factors Society.

Diffrient, N., Tilley, A., Bardagjy, J. (1974). Humanscale 1/2/3. Cambridge, Mass.: MIT Press.

Mandal, A.C. (1976). The Seated Man. Klampenborg: Mandal.

National Institute for Occupational Health and Safety (NIOSH) (1991). Publications on Video Display Terminals (Revised). ANSI/HFS #100-1988. Cincinnati: NIOSH.

Pheasant, S. (1988). Body Space: Anthropometry, Ergonomics and Design. London: Taylor & Francis.

Rodgers, S.H. (1984). Working with Backache. New York: Perinton.

Tadano, P. (1990). A Safety/Prevention Program for VDT Operators: One Company's Approach. Journal of Hand Therapy, 3:64-71.

Yu, C.Y., Keyserling, W.M. (1989). Evaluation of a new work seat for industrial sewing operations. Applied Ergonomics, 20:17-25.

Appendix 9–1

Ergonomic Chair Assessment

Manufacturer: _____ *Model:* _____

Yes-or-No Responses

_____ Does the seat height adjust easily while you are seated?

_____ Does the seat height allow you to rest your feet on the floor?

_____ Does the seat pan tilt forward and back easily while you are seated?

_____ Does the backrest height adjust easily up and down while you are seated?

_____ Does the backrest move forward and backward easily for adjustment while you are seated?

_____ Does the backrest provide firm support to the lower part of your back?

_____ Can you make the adjustments easily without assuming awkward positions?

_____ Are the seat and back contoured and comfortable to adjust to your movements and body shape?

_____ Have you been instructed in how to adjust this chair to fit you properly?

_____ Does the seat support your thighs to just behind the back of the knee?

_____ Do you experience a shock when you touch the chair in cold weather?

_____ Do the seat and back dissipate body heat?

_____ Do you feel supported and comfortable in this chair? If not, why?

_____ Do you like the overall appearance of the chair?

If arms are featured on this chair,

_____ Are you able to get in close to your desk?

_____ Do the armrests allow your elbows to remain comfortably by your side with your shoulders relaxed?

_____ Are the armrests contoured and comfortable?

_____ Are the armrests adjustable in height and distance from your body?

_____ Can the armrests be removed easily without affecting the appearance of the chair?

Manager and Purchaser

_____ Does this chair come in a variety of models to accommodate variations in size of people, yet give a uniform look?

CHAPTER 10

Keyboards

Joe Barry

ABSTRACT

The ergonomic features of various keyboards and the positioning of the keyboard are discussed. The four principal key logics and the reasoning behind the alternatives to the traditional flat keyboard are explored. Recommendations for workplace assessment are made.

My first glance is always at a woman's sleeve. . . . The double line a little above the wrist, where the typewritist presses against the table, was beautifully defined.

Sherlock Holmes
(Sir Arthur Conan Doyle)
(Baring-Gould, 1967, pp. 411-412)

Sherlock Holmes observed that the tools of a person's profession made their marks on the bodies of the users. Since Sherlock's time the computer and its keyboard have been implicated for their ability to make both visible and invisible "marks" on the bodies of their operators. The keyboard has been identified as a culprit in the increasing rise of cumulative trauma disorders (CTD), repetitive strain injury (RSI), or repetitive motion syndrome (RMS) (Tadano, 1990). The monitor has been associated with health risks related to radiation output, eyestrain, and musculoskeletal stress as a result of suboptimal positioning (Leedham, 1991). The fragmentation of work tasks has

157

created occupations in which the keyboard operator keys all day without the relief of other duties (Alden et al, 1972; Yllo, 1962).

This chapter examines the ergonomics of keyboards and monitors to provide therapists with the information needed to make informed recommendations about workplace design. Consideration is given to the biomechanical factors and research regarding positioning and the demands of the computer workstation. The major key logics—QWERTY or Sholes, Dvorak, alphabetic, and Maltron—are examined. Seating, positioning, and other ergonomic considerations of both the keyboard and monitor are discussed. Research on the use of wristrests and their role in the relief of musculoskeletal stress is explored. Finally, recommendations are made on points to be assessed in the evaluation of the fit of a workstation to a worker.

It has been estimated that 50 cents of every worker compensation dollar in the 1990s will be spent on CTD attributed to the use of computers and keyboards. Nearly half of the United States workforce—45 million workers—use keyboards in their work (Horowitz, 1992). In a market analysis by Industrial Innovations, Inc., it was estimated that there are more than 120 million keyboards in the United States and that sales of personal computers have reached 15 million annually. It is estimated that the cost of lost productivity and the cost of treatment of computer-related injuries are about $7 billion a year (Horowitz, 1992). United States Census Bureau figures showed an increase of 1100% in the use of computers in the workplace in the 7 years 1981 to 1987 (Tadano, 1990).

The keyboard is not the only culprit in injuries at the computer. A number of factors are interrelated, such as seating and placement of the keyboard and the monitor.

Seating

The computer workstation is composed of a triangle that consists of the seat, the keyboard, and the monitor (Nusser, 1992). Paper copy, if any, can be considered as either a fourth vertex or as a part of the monitor vertex, as it is in this chapter. Although seating is addressed in Chapter 9, it is discussed briefly herein as one aspect of the work triangle. Changes in any of the components cause changes in the other components of the work triangle. All adjustments and fitting should begin with seating and should be made around correct positioning in and support from the chair (Shute & Starr, 1984).

The optimal posture is an ideal that does not allow for the variation in seating posture in which humans indulge throughout the workday. Kroemer (1988), Mandal (1981), and Verbeek (1991) questioned assumptions about erect posture's being the ideal. In his review of the literature Kroemer (1988, p. 314) observed: " . . . careful examination of the published data indicates no clear benefits of sitting erect as opposed to sitting slumped."

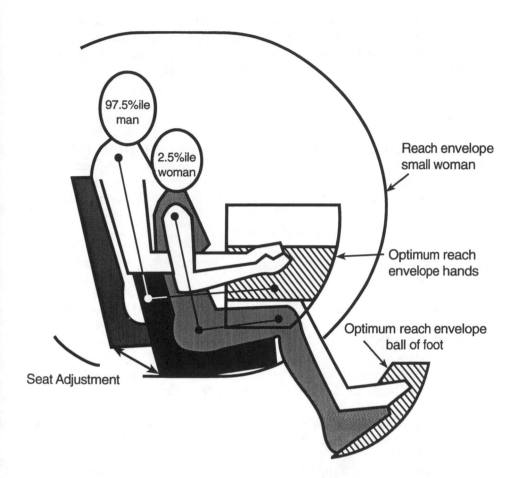

97.5%ile man

2.5%ile woman

Reach envelope small woman

Optimum reach envelope hands

Optimum reach envelope ball of foot

Seat Adjustment

Figure 10–1 Range of adjustment required for workstation. Adapted from Brennan, R.B. (1987). Trencher Operator Seating Positions. Applied Ergonomics, 18(2), 95-102.

The reality is that a seated human moves constantly to relieve pressure under the ischial tuberosities and to rock over the tuberosities to vary the center of gravity and the resultant load on the intervertebral disks (Grandjean et al, 1984; Zacharkow, 1988). Postural change requires adjustability within the workstation. The components of the computer workstation must conform to the needs of the smallest woman in the 5th percentile of anthropometric measurements to the largest man in the 95th percentile (Figure 10–1). The equipment must be easily adjustable by the operator throughout the work period to conform to changes in the seated posture. Grandjean observed that operators who slumped preferred high keyboards because of the relative elevation of the elbow when the operator reclined (Nakaseko et al, 1985).

Changes in posture also affect the operator-screen relationship, necessitating changes in the positioning of the video display terminal (VDT). Other factors such as the use of bifocals affect posture in the seat and necessitate changes in either the seat or the position of the VDT.

Keyboards

A number of keyboards may be classified as ergonomic (Table 10–1). What is an ergonomic keyboard and what benefits there are to using one are open to question. Research findings regarding the arrangement of the keyboard to alleviate the musculoskeletal stress that contribute to CTD must be evaluated.

Keyboards can be categorized as follows:

1. The traditional, or QWERTY, Sholes, or Universal, keyboard (Figure 10–2A)
2. The alphabetic keyboard (Figure 10–2B)
3. Alternative key logic keyboard, such as the Dvorak (Figure 10–2C), Maltron, or virtual-key boards (Figure 10–3)
4. Chord keyboards that require multiple simultaneous keystrokes to enter data
5. Facilitated-communication keyboards designed for users with either physical limitations or communication disorders

Keyboards also can be categorized on the basis of the geometric arrangement of the keys in space. Klockenberg (1926) first suggested the split keyboard to alleviate the ulnar deviation imposed by a flat keyboard. Subsequent developments sought to alleviate stress produced by pronation and wrist flexion by articulating the keyboard. A confusing variety of terms have been used to describe the axes on which the keyboard has been rotated or folded. The clearest description of the three axes in space is as follows:

1. Opening angle (yaw) of 15 to 30 degrees rotation of the left and right halves of the keyboard around a vertical axis to eliminate ulnar deviation of the wrist
2. Lateral angle (roll) or tenting of 30 to 90 degrees of the two halves to reduce or eliminate pronation
3. Slope (tilt) from front to rear to reduce excessive flexion and extension of the wrist (Thompson et al, 1990)

Most keyboards described as ergonomically designed address these geometric features to reduce ulnar deviation and pronation. Some examples of keyboards arranged in space to reduce postural stress are the Maltron (Figure 10–3), Kinesis (Figure 10–4), and Comfort (Figure 10–5) keyboards.

Table 10–1 Ergonomic Keyboards

Manufacturer	Model
AccuCorp, Inc. PO Box 66 Christiansburg, VA 24073 (703) 961-3576	Accukey Ternary chord keyboard
Applied Learning Corporation Box 686 King of Prussia, PA 19406 (215) 688-6866	Importer of PCD Maltron keyboard
ASER Corporation PO Box 92124 Milwaukee, WI 53202	ASER Keyboard
Computability 40000 Grand River, Suite 109 Novi, MI 48050 (313) 477-6720	Adaptive keyboards
Don Johnston Developmental Equipment, Inc. PO Box 639 Wauconda, IL 60084-0639 (800) 999-4660	Adaptive keyboards
Health Care Keyboard Co., Inc. N82 W15340 Appleton Ave. Menomonee Falls, WI 53051 (414) 253-4131	Comfort keyboard
TONY! Ergonomic Keysystems 2332 Thompson Ct. Mountain View, CA 94943 (415) 969-8669	TONY! Keyboard
Industrial Innovations, Inc. 10789 North 90th St. Scottsdale, AZ 85260-6727 (602) 860-8584	DataHand keyboard
Iocomm International Technology 12700 Yukon Ave. Hawthorne, CA 90250 (310) 644-6100	The Wave keyboard
Kinesis Corp. 915 118th Ave. Southeast Bellevue, WA 98005-3855 (206) 455-9220	Kinesis keyboard
Marquardt Switches, Inc. 2711 Route 20 East Cazenovia, NY 13035 (315) 655-8050	Various models
Technical Aids & Systems for the Handicapped Unit 1, 91 Station St. Ajax, Ontario, Canada LIS 3H2 (416) 686-6895	TASH keyboard

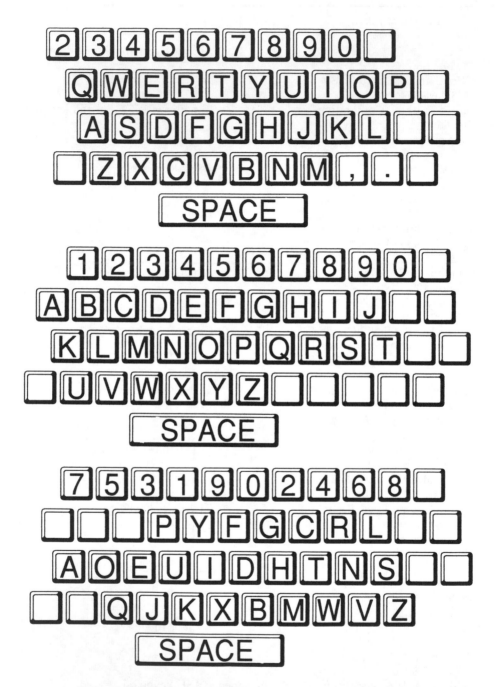

Figure 10–2 Key logic. A. The QWERTY, or Sholes, layout. B. The alphabetic layout. C. The Dvorak (DSK) layout.

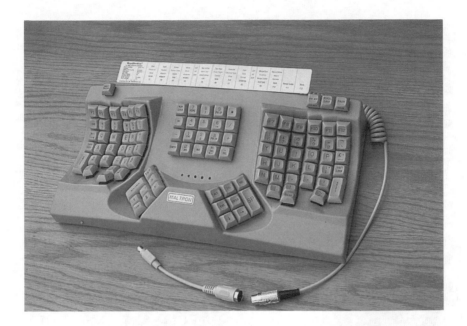

Figure 10–3   Maltron keyboard (courtesy of Applied Learning Corporation).

Sholes, QWERTY, or Universal Keyboard

[QWERTY is] one of the biggest confidence tricks of all time.

Wilfred A. Beeching
Keyboard Historian (Page, 1990)

The standard keyboard evolved as the chance solution to an engineering design problem to fit manufacturing constraints rather than as a design for use (David, 1986). Taken from the first six letters of the top row, it is commonly called the QWERTY keyboard. It is also known as the Sholes or Universal keyboard (Figure 10–2A). The QWERTY keyboard was designed by Christopher Latham Sholes between 1867 and 1872. Sholes was the inventor of the first commercially successful typewriter, which was manufactured by Remington beginning in 1874 (Current, 1954).

Sholes designed for hunt-and-peck typists. Touch typing was not intro-duced until 1888, when the QWERTY keyboard was already 20 years old. In fact, as Hoke (1990) noted, the original makers were not sure who would buy the typewriter and never envisioned touch typing. Touch typing, as it is now

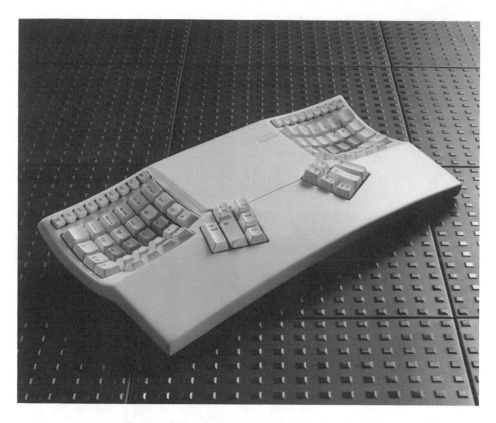

Figure 10–4 Kinesis keyboard (courtesy of Kenesis™ Corporation).

known, with each finger assigned specific keys, was invented by Cuspus Van
Sant and was established in most schools in the United Stated by 1901
(Software Toolworks, 1987).

The QWERTY keyboard was established as the standard after a speed-
typing contest in which the QWERTY keyboard was matched with a keyboard on which separate keys were used for both capital and lower-case
letters. The typist using the latter was a hunt-and-peck typist who used four
fingers. The Sholes keyboard had the advantage of both fewer keys and a shift
key, and the typist had the then-novel idea of memorizing the keyboard and
using all ten fingers. In the early years of the typewriter industry, there never
was a comparison between the Sholes keyboard and other key logics in which
the competitors were equally skilled typists.

Alternatives such as James Bartlett Hammond's Model Two in 1893
offered a curved keyboard with the sequence DHIATENSOR on the home
row. Hammond called this an ideal keyboard because 70% of the words in

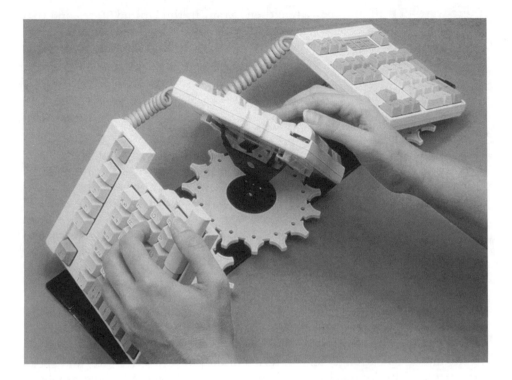

Figure 10–5 Comfort keyboard (courtesy of the Health Care Keyboard Company, Inc.).

the English language can be composed with these ten letters. The Blickensderfer Manufacturing Company also offered a machine with the same arrangement, but by 1896 was offering the Universal model with a QWERTY keyboard. It would appear that after that date the QWERTY keyboard was the standard among the limited options offered by the manufacturers and that the QWERTY method was the standard for typing instruction in the proliferating typing schools.

Alphabetic Keyboards

Beginning with Sholes, whose first keyboard design was alphabetic, the use of an alphabetic keyboard has periodically presented itself as a reasonable design for naive or occasional users (Figure 10–2B). The alphabetic arrangement offers the advantage that little, if any, training is required for the operator to orient to the keyboard. The concept of a naive user is difficult to support at present given the widespread distribution of the QWERTY keyboard for both typewriters and computers. Michaels estimated that in 1971 there were 45 million typewriters then extant in the United States and that one in six Americans used a typewriter for some purpose (Michaels, 1971). The proliferation of the computer since then can only have increased the number of people exposed to the QWERTY keyboard.

The cognitive requirements of an alphabetic keyboard weigh against its use. Hirsch (1970, p. 490) concluded that

> . . . the alphabetical keyboard probably requires, first, a memory search to locate the letter in its approximate or relative alphabetical position, and then a visual search to find the key on the board (where it is situated without regard to the frequency of its use). The combination of the memory plus visual searches may be less efficient than a purely visual search where the probability is high that the visual area first scanned will contain the sought-for letter.

Norman and Fisher (1982) concluded that there was little advantage to considering changing to an alphabetic or Dvorak arrangement because of the minimal differences in productivity. Michaels (1971) found that the most skilled typists showed a large drop in speed when they changed to an alphabetic keyboard and that all groups of less-skilled typists also demonstrated loss of speed in the transition. There were no advantages in output rate, error rate, or speed of typing.

The overall conclusion of all three studies is that there is no advantage to the alphabetic arrangement in terms of output rate, error rate, and speed of learning. The biomechanical demands of the keyboards have not been studied.

Dvorak Keyboard

The general indictment of the "universal" typewriter keyboard . . . remains simply this: its arrangement of key locations has scant reference to the adaptability of your hand skills to the sequence patterns of the written language.

August Dvorak
(Dvorak et al, 1936, p. 217)

In English the most commonly occurring letters are ETAIONSHRLU. Neither the QWERTY nor the alphabetic arrangement places these keys in readily available locations. They require movement ("hurdles") around the keyboard, and these hurdles have not been studied for their effects on the operator. Alternate-key geometry takes as a point of departure this basic observation.

The Dvorak keyboard has experienced a resurgence of interest, as demonstrated by the Apple IIC computer, which is equipped with a switch that instantly converts from QWERTY to virtual Dvorak key logic. (Virtual key logic takes advantage of the fact that the computer key generates an electrical signal whose interpretation can be readily changed. The key is not limited to an unchanging hardware key, physically linked to an arm, with the letter cast on the striking surface, as in the original mechanical typewriter.) Many of the computer typing-tutor programs offer both QWERTY and Dvorak. Why the resurgence of interest in an 80-year-old idea, and is there any advantage to using Dvorak?

In 1936 (1932 in some sources), Dvorak patented the Dvorak Dealey keyboard (Figure 10–2C) (Dvorak et al, 1936), which has since come to be known as the Dvorak Standard Keyboard (DSK). Dvorak was a proponent of motion studies and a student of Frank and Lillian Gilbreth (of *Cheaper by the Dozen* fame). Dvorak et al studied the motions of typists and the task-loading of each finger and analyzed the letter frequency of both single letters and digraphs (such as *t-h*, *e-r*, and *o-n*), in search of the "one best way" (Figure 10–6). The home row of the redesigned keyboard used the same ten letters as Hammond's keyboard (DHIATENSOR), but it eliminated R and added U to that row. The letters were redistributed to facilitate the division of digraphs between hands and fingers to speed input of text. The new home row became AOEUIDHTNS (David, 1986).

The objective of the DSK is to reduce motion by keeping 57.4% of the typing on the home row and balancing the load between the hands with a left-right balance of 37% to 63%. Typists who use the QWERTY keyboard use mostly the keys in the top row of letters with a 49% to 51% hand allocation (Hobday, 1988).

Dvorak observed that the QWERTY keyboard emphasizes use of the left hand in a right-handed world, because the QWERTY keyboard places many of the most common letters and digraphs under the left hand. Perhaps the most egregious placement is that of the letter *a*, the third most commonly used letter in the English language, under the weakest finger for most people—the fifth finger of the left hand (Gould, 1991). This placement requires frequent use of a weak finger and a reach and ulnar deviation that are far from optimal in terms of prevention of injury and productivity. In addition, the keyboard does not account for the congenital linking of the flexor tendons of the fourth and fifth finger in 35% of hands (Hargreaves et al, 1992).

The most common digraphs were designed to be typed with alternate hands for both speed and efficiency of effort (Fox & Stansfield, 1964). Studies of telegraphy have shown that between-hand digraphs are typed faster than same-hand digraphs, and between-finger digraphs are typed faster than same-finger digraphs (Dvorak et al, 1936; Norman & Fisher, 1982). Thirty-four digraphs are used 50% of the time, and 57 digraphs 75% of the time. Only 137 digraphs make up 90% of typed English. Dvorak also examined three- and four-letter combinations in designing his key logic in an attempt to design "machines for men and not men for machines" (David, 1986). (Further

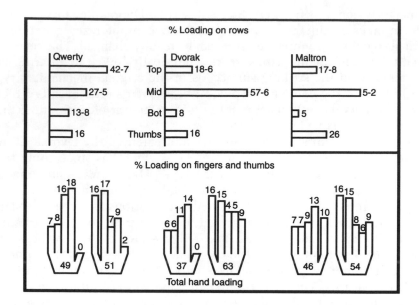

Figure 10–6 Finger and hand loading diagram. Reprinted with permission from Hobday, S.W. (1988). A keyboard to increase productivity and reduce postural stress. In F. Aghazadeh (Ed.), Trends in Ergonomics/Human Factors V. New York: Elsevier Science Publishers.

information about Dvorak keyboards can be obtained from Dvorak International, c/o Trask Office Products, 31 Maple St., Brandon, VT 05733; (802) 247-6747.)

The reasons for the lack of acceptance of the DSK were two simple factors of software and hardware. The software was the pool of typists who were already trained in the use of the QWERTY system and would require retraining. The hardware was the typewriters themselves. The existing typewriters represented a substantial capital investment, and buying new machines or having to maintain stocks of both did not make good business sense. The hardware constraints disappeared with the advent of the computer, which could readily be reprogrammed in how it interpreted key input (i.e., virtual keys). With the higher level and quantity of keying that came with the computer there was both an interest in increased productivity and a new interest in prevention of the CTD that keyboards produced at high rates. The claim that the fingers travel 1.6 km (1 mile) per day on the DSK as opposed to 25.6 km (16 miles) on the QWERTY keyboard has generated a new reason for the interest in the DSK keyboard (Software Toolworks, 1987).

Most of the studies of the DSK are either flawed or limited by their narrow focus. A criticism of most of the studies has been that they were biased because they were performed by Dvorak or the proponents of his keyboard (Rosch, 1984). The most impartial study of the DSK was sponsored by the United States General Services Administration in an attempt to see if retraining typists on the DSK would increase productivity (Strong, 1956). The report concluded that a minimum of 100 hours of instruction and drill (4 hours per day) was required to retrain typists to their previous level of proficiency. The report concluded that recommending the DSK keyboard was not justified.

All of the studies on the DSK limited themselves to two questions. They examined the productivity of workers with the DSK in comparison with the QWERTY and the length of time it took to retrain a typist to a productive level on the DSK. A more relevant area of investigation is the effect of the reduction in motion and balancing of key loads on the incidence of CTD. It would seem that reducing hurdles and stretches and redistributing the most common letters and digraphs to the strongest fingers would reduce the load on the hands and consequently reduce the incidence of microtrauma and the resultant CTD. However, there is no basis in research at this time to support this hypothesis.

PCD Maltron

Named for its inventor, Lillian Malt, this keyboard was invented in 1976 and is manufactured by PCD in England (Figure 10–3). Malt is a skills analyst who trained keyboard operators. Her Maltron keyboard was the first to address not only key logic but also the biomechanics of the human hand and arm. The keyboard is split to prevent ulnar deviation and tipped to eliminate 10 degrees of pronation. Key placement is based on the natural length and arc of the fingers; the design abandons the straight rows of the previous keyboards. The dished configuration of keys is designed around the natural arc of the human hand. It is designed to accommodate the relative lengths of each finger and to allow them to assume a natural, flexed position at rest.

The split keyboard is not a new idea. It was first proposed by Klockenberg in 1926. Rhein-Metal manufactured a split keyboard in the 1930s (Zipp et al, 1983). A more recent split keyboard is the new Apple Adjustable Keyboard, which has been criticized for adjusting only the opening angle and not addressing pronation (Ito, 1993; Markoff, 1993).

The key logic is based on a computer analysis of letter frequency in 1 million English words. The keys were laid out to keep 91% of the most common English letters—ANISFDTHOR—on the home row as compared with 51% for the QWERTY keyboard. The 100 most common words in English can be typed without leaving the home row. The key for the letter *e* is placed under the left thumb because it is the most frequent letter in English, representing 11% of keystrokes. The Maltron keyboard reduces successive use of the same finger 11 times and reduces hurdles 256 times compared with the QWERTY. Hobday (1988) claims that with the QWERTY keyboard as a base of 1.0, the DSK is a 3.27 improvement, and the Maltron is an 11.0

improvement. Hobday is the manufacturer, and an independent analysis has not been done.

Virtual Key Logic

Virtual key logic has become available through the increasing sophistication and computing power of computers. In essence, any key can now be reprogrammed to enter whatever character the user wishes. For example, I use Windows 3.1 as the operating environment and can use the desktop function to remap keys to use foreign letters and scientific or mathematical symbols. Additional fonts are available to expand the possibilities. This is considerably different from the situation in the not-too-distant past, when to work around the default constraints built into a keyboard required the services of a programmer and a search for compatible hardware.

One of the advantages of virtual key logic is the ability to embed keys within the keyboard. The Kinesis keyboard embeds the numbers within the alphabetic keyboard and a shift allows the user to enter numerical rather than alphabetic data (Figure 10–4). Keys can be programmed as special-purpose keys that enter either commonly used functions or macros. Some software is decidedly left- or right-handed in that it requires the use of one hand more than the other to operate the various function keys such as the Control or Alternate key (Harvey, 1991). Virtual keyboards allow the programming of keys or macros to alleviate the demands placed on one hand more than the other.

The most extensive use of virtual keyboards has been developed by a researcher at NEC Corporation to accommodate the four different input modes required in Japan (English, kanji, hiragana, and katagana) (Morita, 1989). To prevent confusion over the varied key functions, a box appears at the bottom of the screen to identify the current key logic.

Chord keyboards

Chord keyboards have been developed to allow rapid input by reducing the number of keys and thus the amount of movement about the keyboard. Chord keyboards get their name from the requirement that two or more keys be depressed simultaneously to encode letters. This is necessitated by the limited number of keys and the need to enter 26 different English letters and ten numbers. Columbo received the first patent for a chord keyboard in 1942 (Noyes, 1983).

The ASCII keyboard, the standard computer keyboard, has 48 data keys. Morita (1989) has suggested that the optimum number for touch typing is 30. Some of the chord keyboards have reduced the number of keys to that of the fingers. There are two-handed keyboards with ten keys and one-handed keyboards with only five keys. The one-handed keyboards are used for data entry or by users with athetoid cerebral palsy or progressive muscular dystrophy (Kirschenbaum et al, 1986).

Ten-key boards can produce 1023 possible chords (Seibel, 1964). Five-key layouts give 31 possibilities (Eilam, 1989), 47 if a sixth key is added for the other thumb (Noyes, 1983). A ternary keyboard has mobile keys. The ternary chord keyboard (TCK) was developed in 1988 by Lawrence J. Langley (Kroemer, 1992). The ternary keys rock forward and backward, giving each key three possibilities for signal generation—forward, centered, and backward. With eight keys the TCK has 6561 possible chords but currently uses only 64. In trials in which users received 3 hours of training and used the keyboard for 10 hours, the users were able to memorize 59 chords and produce 70 characters per minute with a 97% accuracy (Kroemer, 1992).

Chord keyboards are used in specialized applications such as postal sorting and court stenography (Bowen & Guinness, 1965; Conrad & Longman, 1965; Rohmert & Luczak, 1978). There are a limited number of trained users, and most users must be trained on the job. In addition, court stenographers enter data in a form of shorthand that must be deciphered and is prone to error in translation (Seibel, 1964). High rates of entry are possible with stenotype machines, and a skilled operator can produce a verbatim record of spoken English. In fact, a stenotypist was used in a study of voice interactive systems to simulate a computer that used voice entry (Newell et al, 1990; 1991).

Seibel (1964) believes that a good typist can enter almost 100 words per minute (wpm) with a top rate of 150 wpm and that a good stenotypist can enter 200 wpm with possible rates in excess of 300 wpm. Using a short-word vocabulary was found not to influence character keying rate (Schoonard & Boies, 1975) and calls into question the value of systems that require memorization of a shorthand input language. To use a chord keyboard, the user must memorize the chords, which limits the accessibility of the equipment to naive or occasional users. Many of the chord keyboards are unlabeled and are incomprehensible to uninitiated users.

A board with key logic that superficially resembles that of chord keyboards is the DataHand, which uses a finger module around each finger (Figure 10–7) (Adler et al, 1992). The standard 110 keys have been reduced to 54, and the design reduces the hurdles to that of a chord-like layout. Movement of the finger to the front, rear, left, right, and back activates an input signal. Each thumb controls seven functions. The keyboard eliminates float error, which is the most common cause of keyboard error, by eliminating hurdles. The force of activation is reduced, and the repetitive pecking motion is changed to a variety of smaller movements. The change to use of the intrinsic muscles of the hand has not been fully evaluated for its effects on CTD (Ferrell et al, 1992). The molded handrest of the keyboard allows weight-bearing support of the hand and allows use of the arm supports of the chair to support the upper body. It also reduces excess pronation.

The initial release of the DataHand uses a QWERTY key logic so that experienced typists will find each key to be a home key that corresponds to the keys of the home row normally found under that finger. Keys that are

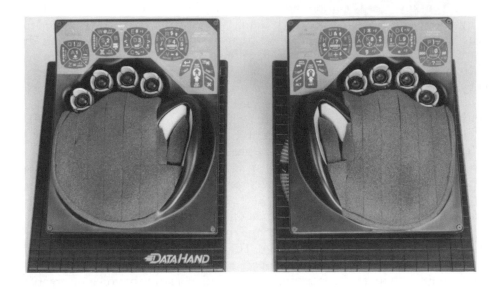

Figure 10–7 DataHand keyboard (courtesy of Industrial Innovations, Inc.).

typically a reach up to the top row are activated by a forward movement of the finger. Only four letters that are diagonal reaches on the QWERTY keyboard—T, Y, B, and N—are not in the "QWERTY" location. Ten hours of practice produced speed equal to the speed with which subjects used a standard keyboard, and users consistently exceeded their speed with a standard keyboard after 20 hours of use (Ferrell et al, 1992). Virtual key logic is used to change the keyboard to three different modes: normal mode, numbers and punctuation mode, and function mode (Figure 10–8). A graphic representation of the three modes is seen on the keyboard rather than on the screen. An additional feature is that each keyboard can use keys to simulate a mouse and can be programmed with different functions, such as coarse and fine movement of the cursor. For computer-aided drafting, one hand can move in the X-Y axis and the other hand in the Z axis.

Adaptive Keyboards

Although a complete review of adaptive keyboards is beyond the scope of this chapter, a brief overview is provided because the technology required to adapt the keyboards is similar to that used in keyboard design in general. Each adaptive keyboard must be customized to the needs of the individual client's disability. Many off-the-shelf keyboards can be adapted through reprogramming keys, virtual key logic, or macros. Some one-handed keyboards such as

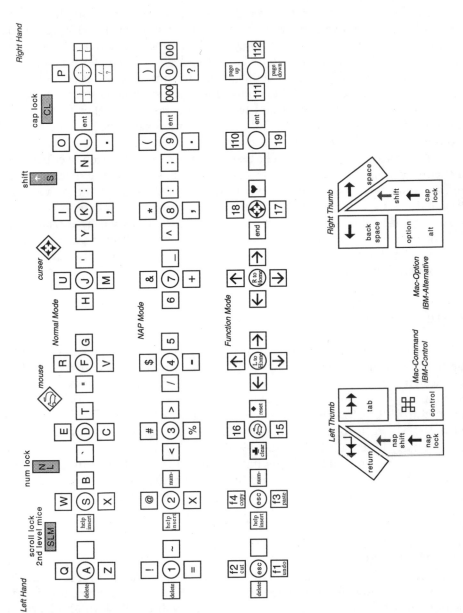

Figure 10–8 DataHand keyboard logic (courtesy of Industrial Innovations, Inc.).

chord keyboards or the left- or right-handed Maltron can be used (Oddo & Angelo, 1992). Special keyboards can be vertically mounted in front of the user and curved to conform to the arc of head movement.

The key logic of adaptive keyboards is sometimes dictated by the limited means of input or movement of the user. Mouthsticks or visors with light-pens are two of many options. The TASH keyboard, manufactured by Technical Aids & Systems for the Handicapped, Inc. (TASH), looks like a target with a bulls-eye. The keys are arranged around the center so that minimal movement of the finger or input device is required. This arrangement assists clients whose range of controlled movement is small and who fatigue easily. Another factor to be considered is that cognitive or perceptual impairments may necessitate adaptations such as pictures or icons on the keys.

Alternative key logic must be tested empirically with each user because a theoretic analysis does not always reflect the best arrangement. In a study of screen-displayed keyboards, Leventhal et al (1991) expected that a square keyboard with a letter-frequency arrangement of the alphabet would be fastest to use followed by a rectangular keyboard and then by a triangular board. They found, however, that the triangle was the fastest to use, possibly because the characters were easy to discriminate and because the layout was more open than that of the other two keyboards.

Postural Constraints

The three historical keyboard arrangements—QWERTY, DSK, and alphabetic—are all flat keyboards shaped more by manufacturing constraints than by design for use. The flat keyboard requires the user to make postural adaptations to conform to the keyboard (Duncan & Ferguson, 1974; Grandjean et al, 1983; Hunting et al, 1981; Zipp et al, 1983). The flat keyboard is also the slowest in the ability of the user to tap, producing a loss in productivity (Creamer & Trumbo, 1960).

These postural adaptations have resulted in the problems associated with keyboard use. As many as one-third of keyboard operators show clinical findings of RSI (Hunting et al, 1981; Kroemer, 1989). The keyboard is not an isolated factor in these injuries but one of many, such as seating, placement of the text and monitor, and the user's history of or predisposition to RSI (Gray et al, 1966; Green et al, 1991; Sauter et al, 1991).

The height of the keyboard is usually the first problem in keyboard placement. The problem faced by furniture designers is that tables must be designed to be low enough to accommodate a 5th-percentile (petite) woman seated with her feet on the floor and high enough to allow thigh clearance under the surface for a 95th-percentile (large) man, according to anthropometric standards (Figure 10–1). No fixed surface is ideal; it is either too high or too low for a large percentage of the population.

The keyboard is usually too high for the operator, who must elevate his or her shoulder girdle to accommodate to the keyboard. This elevation produces a static contraction of the shoulder and back muscles, as confirmed by electromyographic (EMG) studies and reports of discomfort as the keyboard is raised (Life & Pheasant, 1984). A second factor that affects the shoulder girdle is that the hands must be poised over the keys or "hover" without resting on them. The lower key-actuating forces required by computer keyboards than by typewriters have exacerbated this problem and allow no support from the hands and arms. The result is that the trunk provides all the support for the upper body. Good seating becomes critical because of the shifting of support entirely to the spine and abdominal muscles.

Grandjean et al (1984) noted that higher keyboards were preferred by users because the users could lean back at an angle of 97 to 121 degrees. The authors observed that operators do not maintain the ideal posture and typically recline to support the trunk while keying (Grandjean & Hunting, 1977). This is an important factor to keep in mind in the assessment of workstations. The operator cannot maintain comfort in the recommended position and moves throughout the work day.

The reclining posture results in a repositioning of the arms that effectively raises the elbow, resulting in an opening in the angle of the elbow from the recommended 70 degrees to 135 degrees (Human Factors Society, 1988). The conclusion that should be drawn is that the keyboard height not only should be adjustable to fit the range required for 5th-percentile women through 95th-percentile men but also should be readily adjustable during use for the operator to accommodate changing seated postures and obtain relief from static postures (Figure 10–9).

Keyboard elbow supports have been found to be effective in supporting the arms and relieving trapezius contraction and activity (Westgaard & Aarås, 1980). Although trapezius activity increases considerably with the use of wristrests, the rests were preferred by users (Westgaard & Aarås, 1980). Bendix and Jessen (1986) found that wrist supports probably do not present any advantages. Nakaseko et al (1985) found decreased intervertebral disk pressure in the lumbar spine when wristrests were used. This is clearly an issue that requires more research.

Flat keyboards require full pronation of the forearms to place the fingers on the keys (Kroemer, 1972; Rose, 1991). The forearm is limited in pronation to 80 to 85 degrees (Kapandji, 1982; Rose, 1991; Trombly, 1989), 5 to 30 degrees short of a full horizontal position (sources differ). This limitation necessitates abduction and flexion at the shoulder to bring the hand to a full horizontal position (Kroemer, 1972). To approximate the smaller fingers to a horizontal keyboard requires increased finger extension of the fourth and fifth fingers (Ferguson & Duncan, 1974; Rose, 1991).

Lifting the shoulder and elbow places a static load on the shoulder muscles. With key activation forces in the range of 0.6 newtons or less, the

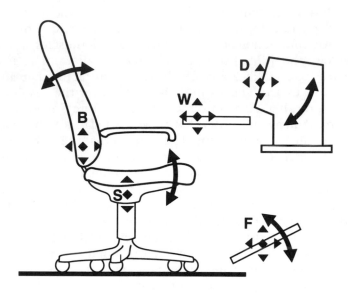

Figure 10–9   Adjustment features of a computer workstation. Adapted from Kroemer, K.H.E. (1988). Ergonomic seats for computer workstations. In F. Aghazadeh (Ed.), Trends in Ergonomics/Human Factors V. New York: Elsevier Science Publishers.

hands cannot support any weight and require static contraction of the arm muscles to hover over the keys.

To fully accommodate to a flat keyboard and the shoulder width, the hand must be deviated to the ulnar side in a wide range (Rose, 1991). This is the basis for split or wing-shaped keyboards. The ". . . split keyboard significantly reduces muscle loading of the trapezius as well as subjective feelings of muscular tension in the shoulder-neck region" (Marek et al, 1991, p. 8).

Finally, keying itself requires a light hovering touch with rapid and repetitive motions. A modest rate of 60 wpm requires 18,000 keystrokes per hour (Brody, 1992). That speed approximates the theoretic limit of 5 to 6 keystrokes per second per finger imposed by the 0.17-second biochemical limit between keystrokes for a single finger (Hobday, 1988). The little research on the effects of this repetitive motion on the hands has been conducted by Gilbert et al (1988) and Garrett (1971). Keying rates can be as high as 50,000 to 200,000 keystrokes per day with an average 3.1 times greater force than the 57 to 95 grams of force required for key activation (Rempel et al, 1991).

Hobday (1988) observed that the onset of CTD can be as rapid as 1 week. The most productive workers are those who make the most repetitive movements and are thus most at risk for RSI. A meta-analysis found strong evidence of a causal relationship between repetitive forceful work and the development of CTD and associated nerve and tendon disorders of the upper extremity (Stock, 1991). In addition, the incidence of CTD may be greatly underreported. In Santa Clara County, the California Department of Health

Services found that the state occupational safety and health officials had 71 reported cases of carpal tunnel syndrome in 1987, while health care providers in the county reported treating just under 4,000 cases, some of which presumably were pre-existing cases (Hembree & Sandoval, 1991).

Somatic complaints have been linked to the work environment. It has been found that job content is a factor in the number of physiologic complaints of VDT operators. Smith et al (1981) found a higher incidence of illness among clerical workers than among professional level staff who also used computers. The use of computers to monitor work output at a keystroke-by-keystroke rate in real time is known as electronic performance monitoring (EPM). EPM is prevalent in monitoring telephone operators and has been found to be related to increases in somatic complaints by monitored employees (Smith et al, 1992; Amick & Smith, 1992; Schleifer, 1992).

Recommendations

In an assessment of the workplace the focus should be on adaptability. Slovak and Trevers (1988) found that ergonomic problems, such as seat adjustment and comfort, outweighed symptomatic problems, such as localized pain, in a ratio of 4:1. Operators will not maintain the preferred posture (Grandjean et al, 1984), so the workstation not only should fit the ideal but also should be readily adjustable throughout the day. Figure 10–9 illustrates the range of adjustments that should be available. They are as follows:

1. The operator's feet should be either on the floor or on a footrest (see Figure 9–3)
2. The scat should be supportive. Chairs should be easily and rapidly adjusted while the user is seated (see Figures 9–1, 9–2)
3. The height of the keyboard should allow the user to adopt an arm angle of 70 to 135 degrees (Human Factors Society, 1988)
4. There should be adequate thigh clearance under the keyboard support
5. The keyboard should reduce keyswitch force, repetition, awkward joint postures, and long durations without recovery time
6. Wrist and arm supports, if appropriate to the task, should reduce static muscular stress
7. Alternate-key geometry should be considered to reduce musculoskeletal stress. Martin (1972) found that once trained on an alternate-key board an operator can switch back and forth in the same manner as a bilingual person who alternates between languages
8. The software or type of data entry should not place excessive loads on the fingers or hands. A redefined keyboard or macros may help redistribute the load
9. Stress, work pace, and musculoskeletal pain should be reduced with micropauses (ie, short or momentary breaks or changes of task)

Conclusion

When evaluating a computer workstation a therapist must examine many factors, such as seating, positioning, adjustability, and alternative interfaces, to reduce musculoskeletal strain. The strength of the computer in the workplace is its adaptability. This adaptability is the key to providing workers with a workplace that is unlikely to produce injury. It is difficult for therapists to keep pace with the rapid changes in the computer industry; contacts within the industry are to be encouraged. Changes caused by advances in computer technology provide the opportunity not only for creative and affordable adaptations but also for the evaluation of new products for potential deleterious effects on users. The likelihood of even greater use of computers in the workplace continues to provide therapists with challenges in adapting a workplace that will not harm the worker.

References

Adler, J., Leonard, E.A., Namuth, T., Hager, M. (1992). Typing without keys. Newsweek, 120 (December 7): 63-64.

Alden, D.G., Daniels, R.W., Kanarick, A.F. (1972). Keyboard design and operation: A review of the major issues. Human Factors, 14:275-293.

Amick, B.C., Smith, M.J. (1992). Stress, computer-based work monitoring and measurement systems: A conceptual overview. Applied Ergonomics, 23: 6-16.

Baring-Gould, W.S. (Ed.) (1967). The Annotated Sherlock Holmes. New York: Potter.

Bendix, T., Jessen, F. (1986). Wrist support during typing: A controlled, electromyographic study. Applied Ergonomics, 17:162-168.

Bowen, H.M., Guinness, G.V. (1965). Preliminary experiments on keyboard design for semiautomatic mail sorting. Journal of Applied Psychology, 49:194-198.

Brody, J.E. (1992). Epidemic at the computer: Hand and arm injuries. New York Times. March 3:B5/8-9.

Brennan, R.B. (1987). Trencher operator seating positions. Applied Ergonomics, 18:95-102.

Conrad, R., Longman, D.J.A. (1965). Standard typewriter versus chord keyboard: An experimental comparison. Ergonomics, 8:177-88.

Creamer, L.R., Trumbo, D.A. (1960). Multifinger tapping performance as a function of the direction of tapping movements. Journal of Applied Psychology, 44:376-380.

Current, R.N. (1954). The Typewriter and the Men Who Made It. Urbana: University of Illinois Press.

David, P.A. (1986). Understanding the economics of QWERTY: The necessity of history. In W.N. Parker (Ed.), Economic History and the Modern Economist (pp. 30-49). New York: Basil Blackwell.

Duncan, J., Ferguson, D. (1974). Keyboard operating posture and symptoms in operating. Ergonomics, 17:651-662.

Dvorak, A., Merrick, N.L., Dealey, W.L., Ford, G.C. (1936). Typewriting Behavior: Psychology Applied to Teaching and Learning Typewriting. New York: American.

Eilam, Z. (1989). Human engineering the one-handed keyboard. Applied Ergonomics, 20:225-229.

Ferguson, D., Duncan, J. (1974). Keyboard design and operating posture. Ergonomics, 17:731-744.

Ferrell, W.R., Knight, L.W., Koeneman, J. (1992). Preliminary test and evaluation of Datahand: A keyboard alternative designed to prevent musculoskeletal disorders and to improve performance. In S. Kumar (Ed.), Advances in Industrial Ergonomics and Safety V (pp. 411-448). New York: Taylor & Francis.

Fox, J.G., Stansfield, R.G. (1964). Digram keying times for typists. Ergonomics, 7:317-320.

Garrett, J.W. (1971). The adult human hand: Some anthropometric and biomechanical considerations. Human Factors, 13:117-131.

Gilbert, B.G., Hahn, H.A., Gilmore, W.E., Schurman, D.L. (1988). Thumbs up: Anthropometry of the first digit. Human Factors, 30:747-750.

Gould, S.J. (1991). The panda's thumb of technology. In S.J. Gould (Ed.), Bully for Brontosaurus: Reflections in Natural History (pp. 59-75). New York: Norton.

Grandjean, E., Hunting, W. (1977). Ergonomics of posture: Review of various problems of standing and sitting posture. Applied Ergonomics, 8:135-140.

Grandjean, E., Hunting, W., Nishiyama, K. (1984). Preferred VDT workstation settings: Body posture and physical impairments. Applied Ergonomics, 15:99-104.

Grandjean, E., Hunting, W., Pidermann, M. (1983). VDT workstation design: Preferred settings and their effects. Human Factors, 25:161-175.

Gray, F.E., Hanson, J.A., Jones, F.P. (1966). Postural aspects of neck muscle tension. Ergonomics, 9:245-256.

Green, R.A., Briggs, C.A., Wrigley, T.V. (1991). Factors related to working posture and its assessment among keyboard operators. Applied Ergonomics, 22:29-35.

Hargreaves, W., Rempel, D., Halpern, N., et al. (1992). Toward a more humane keyboard. CHI '92 Proceedings. Monterey, CA (365-368). Reading, Mass.: Addison-Wesley.

Harvey, D.A. (1991). Health and safety first. Byte, 16:119-127.

Hembree, D., Sandoval, R. (1991). RSI has become the nation's leading work-related illness: How are reporters and editors coping with it? Columbia Journalism Review, 30:41-46.

Hirsch, R.S. (1970). Effects of standard versus alphabetical keyboard formats on typing performance. Journal of Applied Psychology, 54:484-490.

Hobday, S.W. (1988). A keyboard to increase productivity and reduce postural stress. In F. Aghazadeh (Ed.), Trends in Ergonomics/Human Factors V (pp. 321-330). New York: Elsevier.

Hoke, D.R. (1990). Ingenious Yankees: The Rise of the American System of Manufactures in the Private Sector. New York: Columbia University Press.

Horowitz, J.M. (1992). Crippled by computers. Time, October 12, 1992: 70-72.

Human Factors Society (1988). American National Standard for Human Factors Engineering of Visual Display Terminal Workstations (ANSI/HFS Standard No. 100-1988). Santa Monica: Human Factors Society.

Hunting, W., Laubli, T., Grandjean, E. (1981). Postural and visual loads at VDT workplaces. 1. Constrained postures. Ergonomics, 24:917-931.

Industrial Innovations, Inc. (1992). Executive Summary, p. 2.

Ito, R. (1993). Apple goes ergonomic. MacUser, 9 (March):44.

Kapandji, I.A. (1982). The Physiology of the Joints, 5th ed. Vol. 1. Upper Limb. London: Churchill Livingstone.

Kirschenbaum, A., Friedman, Z., Melnik, A. (1986). Performance of disabled persons on a chordic keyboard. Human Factors, 28:187-194.

Klockenberg, E.A. (1926). Rationalisierung der Schreibmaschine und ihrer Bedienung. Berlin: Springer.

Kroemer, K.H.E. (1972). Human engineering the keyboard. Human Factors, 14:51-63.

Kroemer, K.H.E. (1988). Ergonomic seats for computer workstations. In F. Aghazadeh (Ed.), Trends in Ergonomics/Human Factors V (pp. 313-320). New York: Elsevier.

Kroemer, K.H.E. (1989). Cumulative trauma disorders: Their recognition and ergonomics measures to avoid them. Applied Ergonomics, 20:274-280.

Kroemer, K.H.E. (1992). Performance on a prototype keyboard with ternary chorded keys. Applied Ergonomics, 23:83-90.

Leedham, G. (1991). Input/output hardware. In A. Downton (Ed.), Engineering the Human-Computer Interface. London: McGraw-Hill.

Leventhal, L.M., McKeeby, J.W., Mynatt, B.T. (1991). Screen keyboards: An empirical study of the effects of shape and character layout. In H.J. Bullinger (Ed.), Human Aspects in Computing: Design and Use of Interactive Systems and Work with Terminals. New York: Elsevier.

Life, M.A., Pheasant, S.T. (1984). An integrated approach to the study of posture in keyboard operation. Applied Ergonomics, 15:83-90.

Mandal, A.C. (1981). The seated man (homo sedens): The seated work position: Theory and practice. Applied Ergonomics, 12:19-26.

Marek, T., Noworol, C., Wos, H., Karkwowski, W., Krzysztof, H. (1992). Muscular loading and subjective ratings of muscular tension by novices when typing with standard and split-design computer keyboards. International Journal of Human-Computer Interaction, 4:387-394.

Markoff, J. (1993). New keypad for Apple PC is adjustable. New York Times, January 6:D4.

Martin, A. (1972). A new keyboard layout. Applied Ergonomics, 3:48-51.

Michaels, S.E. (1971). Qwerty versus alphabetic keyboards as a function of typing skill. Human Factors, 13:419-426.

Morita, M. (1989). Development of new keyboard optimized from standpoint of ergonomics. In M.J. Smith, G. Salvendy (Eds.), Work with Computers: Organizational, Management, Stress and Health Aspects (pp. 595-603). New York: Elsevier.

Nasaseko, M., Grandjean, E., Hunting, W., Gierer, R. (1985). Studies on ergonomically designed alphanumeric keyboards. Human Factors, 27:175-187.

Newell, A.F., Arnott, J.L., Carter, K., Cruickshank, G. (1990). Listening typewriter simulation studies. International Journal of Man-Machine Studies, 33:1-19.

Newell, A.F., Arnott, J.L., Dye, R., Cairns, A.Y. (1991). A full-speed listening typewriter simulation. International Journal of Man-Machine Studies, 35:119-131.

Norman, D.A., Fisher, D. (1982). Why alphabetic keyboards are not easy to use: Keyboard layout doesn't much matter. Human Factors, 24:509-519.

Noyes, J. (1983). Chord keyboards. Applied Ergonomics, 14:55-59.

Nusser, D.W. (1992). Properly designed work stations pay dividends. Office, 115:26-28.

Oddo, C.R., Angelo, J. (1992). Comparison of two keyboard arrangements for one-handed typists. Work, 2:32-42.

Page, J. (1990). Writing got a lot easier when the old "manual" was new. Smithsonian, 21:54-65.

Rempel, D., Gerson, J., Armstrong, T., Foulke, J., Martin, B. (1991). Fingertip forces while using three different keyboards. Proceedings of the Human Factors Society 35th Annual Meeting, San Francisco (253-255). Santa Monica: Human Factors Society.

Rohmert, W., Luczak, H. (1978). Ergonomics in the design and evaluation of a system for "postal video letter coding." Applied Ergonomics, 9:85-95.

Rosch, W.L. (1984). Keyboard ergonomics for IBMs. PC Magazine, 3:110-122.

Rose, M.J. (1991). Keyboard operating posture and actuation force: Implications for muscle over-use. Applied Ergonomics, 22:198-203.

Sauter, S.L., Schleifer, L.M., Knutson, S.J. (1991). Work posture, workstation design, and musculoskeletal discomfort in a VDT data entry task. Human Factors, 33:151-167.

Schleifer, L.M. (1992). Electronic performance monitoring (EPM). Applied Ergonomics, 23:4-5.

Schoonard, J.W., Boies, S.J. (1975). Short-type: A behavioral analysis of typing and text entry. Human Factors, 17:203-214.

Seibel, R. (1964). Data entry through chord, parallel entry devices. Human Factors, 6:189-192.

Shute, S.J., Starr, S.J. (1984). Effects of adjustable furniture on VDT users. Human Factors, 26:157-170.

Slovak, A.J.M., Trevers, C. (1988). Solving workplace problems associated with VDTs. Applied Ergonomics, 19:99-102.

Smith, M.J., Carayon, P., Sanders, K.J., Lim, S-Y, LeGrande, D. (1992). Employee stress and health complaints in jobs with and without electronic performance monitoring. Applied Ergonomics, 23:17-27.

Smith, M.J., Cohen, B.G.F., Stammerjohn, L.W. (1981). An investigation of health complaints and job stress in video display operations. Human Factors, 23:387-400.

Software Toolworks (1987). Mavis Bacon Teaches Typing! Chatsworth, Calif: The Software Toolworks.

Stock, S.R. (1991). Workplace ergonomic factors and the development of musculoskeletal disorders of the neck and upper limbs: A meta-analysis. American Journal of Industrial Medicine, 19:87-107.

Strong, E.P. (1956). A Comparative Experiment in Simplified Keyboard Retraining and Standard Keyboard Supplementary Training. Washington, D.C.: US General Services Administration.

Tadano, P. (1990). A safety/prevention program for VDT operators: One company's approach. Journal of Hand Therapy, 3:64-71.

Thompson, D.A., Thomas, J., Cone, J., Daponte, A., Markinson, R. (1990). Analysis of the Tony variable geometry VDT keyboard. Proceedings of the Human Factors Society 34th Annual Meeting, Orlando, Fla. (pp. 365-369).

Trombly, C.A. (Ed.) (1989). Occupational Therapy for Physical Dysfunction, 3rd ed. Baltimore: Williams & Wilkins.

Verbeek, J. (1991). The use of adjustable furniture: Evaluation of an instruction programme for office workers. Applied Ergonomics, 22:179-184.

Westgaard, R., Aarås, A. (1980). Static muscle load and illness among workers doing electro-mechanical assemble work. Institute of Work Physiology, Oslo, Norway.

Yllo, A. (1962). The bio-technology of card punching. Ergonomics, 5:75-79.

Zacharkow, D. (1988). Posture: Sitting, Standing, Chair Design and Exercise. Springfield, Ill. Thomas.

Zipp, P., Haider, E., Halpern, N., Rohmert, W. (1983). Keyboard design through physiological strain measurements. Applied Ergonomics, 14:117-122.

PART IV

The Application Process

CHAPTER 11

Ergonomics and Injury Prevention Programs

Carl M. Bettencourt

ABSTRACT

Lifting training, back schools, and ergonomics are methods of injury prevention. These methods are discussed and contrasted. An ergonomic job-analysis case study is presented, and ergonomic controls and their applications are reviewed. An understanding of this information can provide the groundwork for the development and implementation of injury prevention and ergonomic interventions.

Injury prevention and management programs to assist workers in industry are being developed and implemented in a variety of settings. These programs exist within hospital and rehabilitation centers and on the work site itself. A variety of professionals are involved in the planning, delivery, and maintenance of these services. These programs can be based on several different models, methods, and approaches. This chapter provides an overview of three approaches to injury prevention and management—lifting training, back schools, and ergonomic evaluation. The effectiveness of each of these approaches is reviewed and evaluated. An ergonomic job-analysis case study is presented that uses the principles and suggestions described in this book. A comprehensive job-site analysis can be used to provide therapists with the tools and information necessary to initiate an effective injury prevention and management program.

Lifting Training

Approximately one-half of compensable episodes of back pain are related to manual lifting (Snook, 1988). Over the years programs have been instituted to teach workers to lift safely using the principles of bending the knees, keeping the back straight, lifting with the leg muscles, holding loads close to the body, and pivoting the feet instead of twisting the trunk. Lifting training is based on the assumption that back injuries are caused by inadequate lifting techniques and therefore that lifting injuries can be prevented by teaching people the safe and correct method of lifting. Safe lifting programs usually involve a review of the anatomic and physiologic features of the spine, the causes of back pain, and basic ergonomic principles.

Several studies have been conducted over the years to validate the effectiveness of lifting training as a means to prevent injuries in the work place. The concept of bending the knees rather than the back has been advocated since the 1930s. However, since that time there has been no overall reduction in the number of injuries attributed to lifting and handling (Pheasant, 1991). Snook (1978) conducted a study of training as a means to prevent industrial back injuries. He compared programs that provided safe-lifting instruction and those that did not and found no evidence that organizations that provided safe-lifting programs had fewer injuries. Studies have noted the effectiveness of safe-lifting programs in reducing injury rates and lost time on the job, but these studies have been poorly documented and made no claims of scientific validation of positive outcomes. Injury statistics taken over an 8-year period for nursing staff in the Canterbury and Thanet area of southeast England indicate a dramatic decrease in injury rates after the implementation of an injury prevention program. The improvement lasted approximately 18 months, after which the injury rates climbed to the pre-program rate. In a study of lifting technique and its relation to reduction in risk, a group of nurses trained in the conventional manner was compared with a group trained by a method that emphasized a problem-solving approach based on ergonomic and biomechanical principles. Although the latter group demonstrated considerable improvement in client-handling technique, a follow-up study showed no statistically significant differences between the two groups in regard to back injuries or back pain (Pheasant, 1991).

Two studies reported a 65% and a 70% reduction in back disability after workers were trained in safe-lifting principles. The results of these two

TABLE 11–1   Questions About Lifting Programs (Pheasant, 1991)

- Are the techniques taught biomechanically correct?
- Do the trainees learn and remember the procedures they have been taught and acquire the necessary skills?
- Are the techniques that have been learned transferred to the working situation? Do they become part of the trainee's instinctive movement behavior?
- Does the training program cover a wide range of practically relevant lifting and handling tasks?
- Are there hidden disadvantages to the correct lifting technique that prevent it from being applied in the workplace?
- Do the practical constraints of the working situation or the nature of the load prevent the student from using the correct lifting technique?
- Is the weight of the load beyond reasonable limits? Is the load inherently unsafe for some other reason (bulk, instability, poor grip)?
- Is the overall physical workload beyond reasonable limits?
- Are lifting and handling the principal causes of back pain in the working population concerned?
- Is the social ethos of the workplace conducive to the maintenance of safe working practices?

studies have been questioned because controls were not used and the studies were not of sufficiently long duration to provide statistically significant results. The National Institute for Occupational Safety and Health (NIOSH) questions the value of safe-lifting training because no controlled studies have demonstrated a drop in injury rates after training (Snook, 1988). Pheasant presented a list of questions to ask about a lifting program in the workplace and implied that successful lifting programs are the exception rather than the rule (Pheasant, 1991) (Table 11–1).

Back Schools

Back schools were originally designed as treatment—to educate patients who were already suffering back pain (Snook, 1988). They are currently being used to educate workers about the prevention and management of back pain. Back schools are comprehensive injury prevention programs that teach more than basic lifting training. They function to educate the worker in all aspects of back care. Back schools encourage the active involvement and responsibility of each participant in a program to reduce back injuries. They are designed to address several areas to improve health and reduce injuries in and out of the workplace. These injury prevention programs involve a variety of components, including the anatomic and physiologic characteristics of the spine, causes of back injuries, posture, exercise, prevention, ergonomics, proper body mechanics, first-aid, activities of daily living, vocational guidance, job simulation, job-site instruction, nutrition, and stress management. Back schools use techniques such as education, group participation, slide or videotape presentations, poster presentations, and printed literature to educate participants and encourage behavioral changes at work and at home. Many back schools also train and enlist the support of managers and supervisors on the job site. This allows managers to be aware of the importance of the information being presented and ensures follow-through of learned principles on a day-to-day basis. Back schools also encourage periodic review of the content presented, which encourages long-term compliance.

The effectiveness of back schools in reducing injuries in the workplace has been demonstrated in several studies. A controlled longitudinal field study was carried out at a bus company in the Netherlands to assess the cost-effectiveness of a back school. The results noted a reduction in absenteeism by a least 5 days per year per employee (Versloot et al, 1992). Clients with acute back problems from the Volvo works at Goteborg, Sweden, who participated in a back school were able to return to work sooner than a control group who underwent conventional physical therapy (Pheasant, 1991; Snook, 1988). Moffett et al (1986) compared clients with chronic back pain who attended a back school with a control group who were treated with exercise only. The authors reported that both treatments were effective in the short term; however, only the patients who participated in the back school showed long-term improvement with respect to pain and functional disability (Moffett et al, 1986). Participants from a rheumatology center in Holland were assigned to a back school or a control group. No statistically significant differences in reported pain or spinal mobility were observed in either group after 1 year. The authors concluded that a back school should be used in the early phases of back pain. The Southern Pacific Company reported a 22% reduction in the number of workers treated for low-back pain and a 43% decrease in days of work lost after 2 years of using the California Back School in a preventive program for its 30,000 workers. PPG Industries reported a 70% reduction in the number of injuries and a 90% reduction the cost of injuries after 2 years of using the Atlanta Back School in a preventive program for its 2000 employees (Snook, 1988). The Spine Center in Dallas reported a 40% decrease in days lost from work the year after the introduction of back schools in eight industries (Snook, 1988).

An abundance of literature supports the effectiveness of back schools in terms of reduced injury rates and time lost from work (Anderson, 1989; Burrous, 1988; Industry Safety Tips, 1985; Isernhagen, 1988; Schwartz, 1990; Stulz, 1990). However, many of the studies cited lacked controls to enable statistical comparison. This lack of comparison data may cause one to question the effectiveness of back schools, but the value of these programs appears to be encouraging.

Ergonomics and Injury Prevention

The science of ergonomics is approximately 40 years old. It was founded by a group of British anatomists, physiologists, psychologists, and engineers who advocated a multidisciplinary, scientific approach to the study of work efficiency. A similar discipline emerged in North America and was called human factors. At present both names are associated with the science of ergonomics (Pheasant, 1991).

Ergonomic approaches to injury are being used as a method of injury prevention. Ergonomic injury prevention intervention in industry focuses on fitting the job to the worker. This approach studies the job and variables that may place a worker at risk for injury. A job analysis functions as the basis for job modifications. Factors to modify include the workstation, tools, equipment, the job description, and the work environment. The job analysis is a key component of this interventional method. Appendixes 1, 2, and 3 at the end of this book present three job-analysis protocols. These protocols address a variety of factors inherent in a worker's job that should be used to identify areas that may interfere with maximal function.

Industry is documenting the effectiveness of incorporating an ergonomic approach to injury prevention programs (Armstrong, 1986; Bureau of National Affairs, 1988; Buckle & Stubbs, 1989; Jackson, 1991; Joyce, 1988; Lutz & Hansford, 1991; MacLeod et al, 1990; McReynolds, 1991; Moretz, 1989; Pheasant, 1991; Schumacher, 1990). This literature illustrates the effectiveness of ergonomic intervention and describes benefits in terms of decreased employee sick leave, low injury rates, reduced worker compensation payments, early return to work after injuries, increased worker satisfaction, and overall financial savings.

The ergonomic approach, fitting the job to the worker, can be expanded to fitting the worker to the job. Pheasant (1991) presents a model for this approach. Fitting the person to the job involves selection and screening, skills training, safety training, fitness training, health education, back-care education, and stress management. Fitting the job to the person involves work design, safety engineering, environmental control, and organizational change (Pheasant, 1991). These two approaches can be combined for an effective injury prevention program in the workplace. This complementary approach is illustrated in the use of the ergonomic team. This team includes health care providers, health and safety personnel, managers, and employees (Gross,

1990; Haag, 1992; Kazutaka, 1989; Lutz & Hansford, 1987; McCasland, 1992; Travers, 1992) (see Appendixes 1, 2, and 3.)

Discussion

All three approaches to the control of injuries in the workplace—training, back schools, and ergonomic modification—appear to have merit. However, none has been proved to be conclusively superior for reducing injuries in all workplaces. Each of these injury prevention and management programs is effective in some way. There appears to be evidence to account for various levels of cost-effectiveness, reductions in injury rates, and reductions in lost time.

Lifting training in itself does not appear to be the answer to reducing injuries in the workplace. There is little evidence to support the effectiveness of this approach. Reports in the literature contain a lack of statistical validation of positive outcomes and show that the duration of the effectiveness of this training method is short. The problem may exist not in the training of safe lifting techniques but in workers' compliance with the recommendations (Schwartz, 1990; Snook, 1988). The degree of managerial support for this intervention and the workers' perspective are areas to be considered with this approach. Most workers have established patterns and habits for performing work, which makes lifting training difficult to enforce. Training workers in safe lifting may be more effective for employees with a history of back pain because they are more likely to comply than are other employees (Snook, 1988).

Back schools introduce a wide spectrum of variables to consider in injury prevention and management. A fundamental feature in this approach is the inclusion of the trainee as an active participant. This approach encourages the trainee to take responsibility for injury prevention and management. This approach is supported in a variety of studies that document the effectiveness of back schools in reducing back pain and disability. Some studies on the effectiveness of back schools include statistical evidence of their benefit. Most of these studies were performed in hospitals, where it may be easier to control the conditions than in industrial settings. In addition, the studies did not include people who did not have back pain. Despite the lack of control data, the financial savings to industry may justify the use of back schools as a valid injury prevention tool. The ergonomic approach centers on evaluating the job site and modifying jobs to accommodate the working population. A considerable number of studies in the literature support this method of injury prevention. The ergonomic team comprises experts in several disciplines who provide ergonomic evaluation and recommendations for modification and who provide training, such as lifting programs and back schools. The approach is based on the idea that no single method of injury prevention is effective in reducing injuries. This combination of approaches (ergonomic design, job analysis, and training) is supported in the literature (Bell, 1991; Jackson, 1991; MacLeod, 1990; Snook, 1988).

One of the most effective components of the ergonomic team approach to injury prevention in the workplace is the education and collaboration of managers, unions, and practitioners. The use of an ergonomic team appears to be effective in addressing the multidimensional nature of injuries in the workplace because it considers many of the variables that predispose workers to injuries.

It is important to consider the worker's characteristics and the interaction between machine (job) and worker. The protocols for job analysis (Appendixes 1, 2, and 3) present a variety of areas to be considered. Central to each of these approaches is the activity breakdown and analysis of each job function. This process serves to identify the components and characteristics of each job. It can provide the basis for functional job descriptions, job modifications, and injury prevention programs. The following case study presents an ergonomic job analysis and recommendations to address identified stressors.

Case Study

The job analysis was done at a Fortune 500 company that manufactures medical products and measuring tools and that uses computers to design equipment, including cars, and to produce photographic animation. The subject of the analysis (the worker) was the company nurse.

Worker Attributes

Job Title: Certified Occupational Health Nurse (COHN)
Name: Marion
Age: 41 years
Height: 5 feet, 3 inches (160 cm)
Weight: 200 pounds (91 kg)
Hand Dominance: Right

Subjective Job Description

Marion is the nurse for a Fortune 500 company. She is employed 40 hours per week. She works Monday through Friday from 7:00 a.m. to 3:30 p.m. She is a salaried employee and is able to take a 30- to 60-minute daily lunch break. She is also able to take intermittent breaks throughout the day. Her job responsibilities are varied. They include coordination of the employee disability program, worker compensation claims, and the direction of the medical emergency response team. This response team includes groups of volunteer employees who are taught cardiopulmonary resuscitation (CPR) and first aid. Marion is responsible for four buildings throughout the city, which house a total of 11,000 employees. She is also in charge of the company's fitness center and coordinates wellness and fitness programs for the employees. In addition to these responsibilities, Marion reports spending an average of 5 hours a day involved in computer-related work. She reports that this work can occasionally be required for an entire 8-hour work day on a continuous basis.

Marion reports that the fluorescent lighting in her office can be a problem. She describes blinding headaches at the end of the day and pain across her shoulders, neck, and wrists on days when she is involved with intensive computer work. She has addressed this problem by turning off one of the overhead fluorescent lights, adjusting the window blinds, and equipping her computer keyboards with 18 × 2 inch (46 × 5 cm) wristrests. These measures have decreased but not eliminated her symptoms.

Work Pace

Marion is not expected to operate on a set schedule in terms of rigid production standards; however, her job pace has changed considerably in the past few months. Because of budget cuts at the company, the nursing staff has been decreased from two nurses to one. Marion is currently expected to "pick up the slack" and perform the job of two people. She is also concerned with the stability of her own position and the possibility of additional staff cuts, which could affect her job.

Despite this situation, Marion is generally able to structure her time and allow for rest during her work day. She is free to take spontaneous pauses during intensive computer work and briefly get up and stretch. Disguised pauses (Grandjean, 1990) allow Marion to continue her work yet vary her position by moving from one room to another or changing position to perform another task related to the job at hand. These pauses occur with phone calls, interruptions from employees, and meetings.

Mental Workload and Psychosocial Environment

Because the nursing staff has been decreased from two to one, Marion's job demands have essentially doubled. This situation has decreased the number of rest periods Marion takes and potentially increases the amount of stress she may experience. Marion reports this stress is partially due to the absence of a second nurse with whom to consult for decision making. This situation eliminates the support of a peer with a similar background. Marion also finds herself listening to other employees who feel pressured by managers to improve their overall performance and production. These concerns are coupled with the fears employees express about layoffs and with Marion's concerns about her own job security.

Description of Physical Work Environment

Marion's workstation, which includes a video display terminal (VDT), is located in an office that measures 8 × 17 feet (2.4 × 5.2 m). The room is fully carpeted with a low-pile gray carpet. The walls are painted off-white with a matte finish. The room is illuminated with overhead fluorescent light fixtures. There is also a 4 × 8 foot (1.2 × 2.4 m) window equipped with adjustable blinds. The light that enters through this window is shaded by an outside overhang and several trees, which filter the incoming light. According to Grandjean (1990), the colors of different work surfaces should be of similar brightness; black and white contrasts should be avoided; and a matte rather than a glossy finish should be used. Light fixtures positioned directly overhead can dim the characters on the VDT screen with blurred reflections. VDT workstations should be placed at a right angle to windows to avoid direct glare.

Marion's office is quiet and there are no auditory distractions. Despite this quiet atmosphere, Marion is not isolated because her office is adjacent to the fitness center. This situation provides Marion with a steady source of social stimulation from employees entering and leaving the fitness center. Marion is able to close her door to minimize this distraction. The office climate is temperature-controlled with comfortable conditions that can be manually adjusted as necessary. Marion's job requires no lifting or material-handling of considerable resistance or frequency.

Workstation Design

Marion's workstation is composed of two desks in an L-shaped configuration. The desk that holds the computers is at a right angle to the window, which is on the other side of the room. These desks are both cream-colored with a simulated-oak surface. Both desks are 60 inches (152 cm) wide, 30 inches (76 cm) deep, and 29 inches (74 cm) high.

An ergonomic workstation should accommodate most people working on a given job, not merely an average person. A suggested workstation height is 25.6 to 32.4 inches (64 to 81 cm) (Putz-Anderson, 1991). Marion's workstation height falls within this recommendation, but her working posture indicates that her keyboard may be too high. The ergonomic design specification for depth under the work surface for seated workers is 20.4 to 26.4 inches (51 to 66 cm) (Putz-Anderson, 1991). Vertical and horizontal leg room under an office desk should allow for plenty of leg movement. It is advantageous if workers can cross their legs without difficulty (Grandjean, 1990). Marion's workstation depth is greater than the specification and offers ample room for lower-extremity clearance.

One of Marion's desks is parallel to and against a wall. It holds one computer and two monitors, two keyboards, a 11 × 15 inch (28 × 38 cm) paper holder, a mouse, a tracking ball, and several books. Both monitors are positioned at angles on opposite corners of the desk. The monitor in the left corner measures $20 \times 14 \times 11.5$ inches ($51 \times 36 \times 29$ cm) and sits on top of its drive computer. The larger monitor, which measures $19 \times 20 \times 15$ inches ($48 \times 51 \times 38$ cm), is angled on the right corner. Its drive is under the desk. Both keyboards, one measuring 19×8 inches (48×20 cm), the other measuring 20.5×7 inches (52×18 cm), are positioned at angles parallel to both VDTs. The keys require minimal tactile pressure to activate and emit an audible click when depressed, which serves as a source of auditory feedback with operation. The keyboards are equipped with wristrests measuring 18×2 inches (46×5 cm), which sit in front of them. The keyboards are 0 to 6 inches (0 to 15 cm) from the front of the desk because of their angled position. One of the computer systems is equipped with a mouse and the other with a tracking ball.

Marion reports greater ease of operation with the tracking ball because it remains stationary and does not require wrist and arm movement, as is necessary with mouse operation. She finds the tracking ball more comfortable because her hand rests in a neutral position and does not have to maintain an opposing force between the ulnar and radial aspects of the hand, which is characteristic of mouse operation. This minimizes hand cramping.

Beneath the desk that holds the monitors are a laser printer, a wastebasket, and the drive for one computer. This congested arrangement prevents clearance for Marion's legs when she sits at her computer. The other desk is perpendicular to the right corner of the computer desk. It holds a telephone in the top left-hand corner 18 inches (46 cm) from the front of the desk. The rest of the surface is used for work space. This desk is equipped with two 15 $\times$ 18 inch (38×46 cm) drawers on either side for storage and an unobstructed space to accommodate Marion's legs when she sits (Figure 11–1). Across from the desk that holds the telephone and beneath the window is a lateral file cabinet that is 3 feet (91 cm) wide, 15 inches (38 cm) deep, and 30 inches (76 cm) high. It is the same color as the desks.

Marion sits in a blue upholstered office chair with a contoured backrest and seat surface pads 3 to 4 inches (8 to 10 cm) thick. The seat has a slight hollow with the front edge turned upward. The height of the chair can be adjusted with a knob that is underneath the seat pan. It is also equipped with a five-arm base, casters, and a back pad angled at 105 degrees. This backrest supports Marion up to her shoulder level. The padding of the backrest is convex at the level of the lumbar spine and concave at thoracic level. The backrest has an adjustable inclination, which Marion controls by leaning back as far as 120 degrees and allowing it to return by spring action. The height of the backrest can be adjusted with a knob at its base. The chair has adjustable plastic arm supports with rounded edges.

Several studies have yielded the following desirable qualities for office chairs (Grandjean, 1990) (see Chapter 9):

1.   A design for traditional office work and use of VDTs

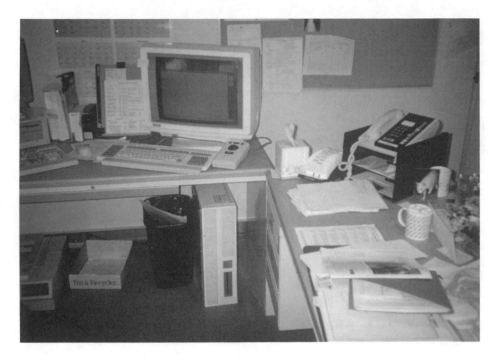

Figure 11–1 Composition of a workstation.

2. Allowance for forward and reclined sitting postures
3. Adjustable backrest inclination and lockable inclination when the desired position is obtained
4. A backrest height of 18.8 to 20.4 inches (48 to 52 cm) above the seat surface. The upper portion of the backrest should be slightly concave. The backrest should be 12.2 to 14.1 inches (32 to 36 cm) wide
5. A backrest with a well-formed lumbar support
6. A seat surface 15.7 to 17.7 inches (40 to 45 cm) across and 14.9 to 16.5 inches (38 to 42 cm) from front to back and with a slight hollow, the front edge of which contours upward
7. Footrests that prevent short people from sitting with hanging feet
8. A height that adjusts from 14.9 to 21.2 inches (38 to 54 cm)
9. Swivel casters or glides, a five-arm base, and user-friendly controls.

Worker-Machine Interaction

When Marion works with the computer monitors, she assumes a stooped and twisted posture. Although the desk provides ample knee clearance, Marion does not take advantage of it because of the equipment stored under the desk.

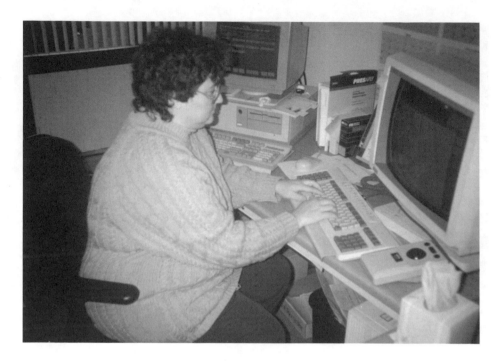

Figure 11–2 Worker at a workstation.

As a consequence, she cannot position her chair close to the work surface, and she compensates by assuming a forward-flexed trunk posture. In this position, Marion cannot fully benefit from the back support of the chair. Her back muscles remain in static contraction to allow her to assume this unsupported position, which increases the likelihood of fatigue and muscle soreness (Figure 11–2).

When Marion sits at the keyboard to enter data into the computer, her line of vision to the center of the monitor is 10 degrees below the horizontal plane for the smaller screen and 20 degrees below horizontal for the larger screen. The preferred line of vision is an average of 10 to 15 degrees below the horizontal plane (Grandjean, 1990). These screen measurements indicate that the middle of the second screen is 5 degrees lower than the preferred line of vision. This low line of vision may partially account for the discomfort Marion feels when she works for a prolonged period of time at the computer. Marion's computer monitors are 22 inches (56 cm) away from her. Most computer operators tend to place their screens 28 to 37 inches (71 to 93 cm) away from themselves for comfortable viewing, although no explanation can be found for this preference (Grandjean, 1990). Marion's proximity to the screens also may account for her discomfort after prolonged computer work.

Marion is subject to eyestrain because of glare from the overhead lighting and the light that comes through the window. The glass of a screen reflects about 4% of incident light. It also reflects office surroundings, such as lights, the keyboard, and the operator's image (Grandjean, 1990).

When Marion is operating the keyboard, she receives limited benefit from the wristrests because of the angle that places the board 0 to 6 inches (0 to 15 cm) from the front of the desk. Marion is able to support only the hand that is on the side with a 6-inch (15-cm) clearance at the distal palmar region. The other wrist has minimal support because Marion's hand hangs off the edge of the desk. Marion's inability to get close to her work, because of the objects under the desk, makes it difficult for her to support her elbows on the armrests of the chair. This affords her little arm support, and her shoulder girdle must compensate for this lack of support by contracting to maintain her arms in a suspended position. This static muscle contraction increases the likelihood of shoulder and neck soreness.

The casters on Marion's chair do not roll smoothly because of the friction from the carpeted floor. This produces resistance when Marion attempts to push her chair from one desk to the other, answer the telephone, reposition herself from one computer monitor to the other, or retrieve materials from the filing cabinet.

Marion uses the telephone frequently during the course of her workday. To answer the telephone when she is working at the computer terminals, Marion must push the chair from one table to the other and reach for the receiver. This maneuver is impeded by the difficulty of moving the chair on the carpet. This repetitive reaching, stretching, and bending of the trunk to answer the telephone that is located beyond her reach when she is seated before the computer terminals probably precipitates Marion's muscle fatigue and soreness. Reaching too far leads to excessive trunk movement and increases the likelihood of pain in the back and shoulders (Grandjean, 1990) (see Chapter 9).

Remediations

Stressor: Screen glare

Reflected glare may be attributed to the location of the computer monitors on the desk top. The location of the screen produces glare from the overhead fluorescent light fixtures as well as from the window to the right of the workstation.

Recommendations

1. Turn off some of the overhead light fixtures and adjust the window blinds. Marion had already addressed this problem
2. Position the VDT so that the overhead fixtures are parallel to and on either side of the VDT

3. Equip the screens with adjustable stands. This enables the screens to be manually adjusted at angles that eliminate reflected glare
4. Equip the screens with filters to minimize reflected glare

Stressor: Headaches and irritated vision

Headaches and irritated vision may be partially attributed to the reflected glare. Another cause may be Marion's proximity to the monitors.

Recommendation

Move the desk 6 to 12 inches (15 to 30 cm) away from the wall to provide enough space to move the monitors farther back on the corners of the desk.

Stressor: Distance from keyboard and angle of body to desk

Marion is unable to get close to her work and position her feet and legs beneath the VDT workstation because this space is used as a storage area for a printer, a computer drive, and a wastebasket.

Recommendations

1. Clear the area beneath the desk. Place the printer and drive on a table to the left of the workstation and place the larger monitor on top of the drive. Marion will then be able to place her legs under the desk and position herself closer to the computer. She then will be able to use the back and arm supports of the chair and eliminate the stooped posture
2. Attend an education session on the importance of workstation posture to promote proper body alignment and minimize fatigue and muscle soreness
3. Adjust the height of the chair to allow a comfortable reach to the keyboard. Use a footrest if adjusting the height of the chair does not allow a comfortable foot position on the floor.

Stressor: Lack of wrist and elbow support

Because of the proximity of the keyboards to the front of the desk, Marion does not have ample wrist support despite the wrist support bars positioned in front of the keyboards. These wrist support bars actually decrease the space available at the edge of the desk. In addition, the objects stored beneath the desk make it impossible for Marion to get close to the desk. As a consequence, Marion must bend forward and cannot benefit from the chair's arm supports, so her shoulders must support the weight of her arms.

Recommendations

1. Remove the objects under the desk. This allows Marion to get close to the desk, making it possible for her to use the arm supports of the chair
2. Provide more space at the front of the desk by moving the desk away from the wall and moving the monitors back
3. Affix a drawer-like platform to the front of the desk to hold the keyboards and provide wrist and forearm support

Stressor: Repetitive reaching and twisting for telephone

Marion's telephone, located to the right of her VDT on the second desk, is beyond her comfortable reach. Marion is forced to bend, reach, and twist to pick up the telephone receiver.

Recommendations

1. Position the telephone on the second desk within reach
2. Position the telephone on the first desk within reach
3. Equip the workstation with a portable headset to eliminate manual telephone use.

Stressor: Chair does not easily move on carpeted surface

The casters of the chair do not roll freely because of friction from the carpeted floor.

Recommendation

Install a lucite or plastic mat on floor under the chair to facilitate movement over the carpeted surface.

Stressor: Workload and psychosocial issues

Marion reports an increased workload since the nursing staff has been decreased from two to one. She is also concerned that her position will be eliminated. In addition, other employees confide in her about feelings of being overworked and about their fears of layoffs.

Recommendations

1. Attend a seminar on stress-management techniques to address and manage concerns and to provide other employees with this information
2. Consult a bibliography of literature on stress management and tools for coping with job-related stress
3. Seek a support group or counselor who specializes in job-related stress
4. Take additional rest periods throughout the work day to compensate for increased work demands.

Tools for Job Analysis

The case study presents one approach to ergonomic job analysis. Potential ergonomic stressors were identified and suggestions offered to allow the worker to interact with her workstation with a greater degree of comfort. Slides provided a means to assist with the analysis and to justify recommendations. Slides or a videotape can be useful data-collection tools for accurate identification of stressors on the job. These tools allow visual documentation, which helps with subsequent reviews of a particular job. Specific stressors may not be apparent at the first viewing but may manifest themselves on subsequent study of the slides or videotape.

A useful tool for job analysis is the *Dictionary of Occupational Titles.* This manual provides a general description of specific jobs and can assist in identifying the various aspects of the job to be evaluated.

Application of Recommendations

Recommendations to address identified stressors on a particular job are referred to as administrative controls and engineering controls. The correct selection and application of these controls to situations that have the potential for producing stress can help alleviate or eliminate adverse work conditions.

Administrative Controls

Administrative controls involve the selection and training of workers for a particular job. The concept of administrative controls parallels Pheasant's description of fitting the person to the job (Pheasant, 1991). This selection can include a clinical evaluation or strength and endurance testing specific to a particular job. The training of workers includes skills, safety, and fitness training for a specific job. It also includes health and back-care education. Administrative controls include measures to reduce the frequency, duration, and severity of exposures to stressors in the work environment. Administrative controls for the meat-packing industry are as follows (United States Department of Labor, 1991):

1. Reducing the total number of repetitions per employee by decreasing production rates and limiting overtime work
2. Providing rest pauses to relieve fatigued muscle-tendon groups. The length of time needed depends on the overall effort and total cycle time of the task
3. Increasing the number of employees assigned to a task to alleviate severe conditions, especially in lifting heavy objects

4. Using job rotation with caution and as a preventive measure, not as a response to symptoms. The principle of job rotation is to alleviate physical fatigue and stress on a particular set of muscles and tendons by rotating employees among other jobs that use different muscle-tendon groups. If rotation is used, job analyses must be reviewed by a qualified person to ensure that the same muscle-tendon groups are not used in the different tasks
5. Providing sufficient numbers of standby or relief personnel to compensate for foreseeable upset conditions on the job, such as loss of workers
6. Enlarging jobs to allow employees to perform more parts of a job as opposed to one specific, repetitive task. The physiologic principle of job enlargement is similar to that of job rotation in that it serves to alleviate physical fatigue and stress on a particular set of muscles and tendons
7. Providing a preventive maintenance program for mechanical and power tools to verify that equipment is in proper working order and within the manufacturer's specifications. This may include vibration monitoring
8. Performing maintenance regularly and whenever workers report problems. Sufficient numbers of spare tools should be available to facilitate regular maintenance
9. Providing a knife-sharpening program. Sharp knives should be readily available
10. Providing housekeeping programs to minimize slippery work surfaces to prevent falls.

Engineering Controls

Engineering controls are a method of modifying a particular workstation, tool, or work method. These controls are designed to eliminate physical fatigue and stress caused by awkward postures, excessive exertion, and repetitive motions in the workplace. The following is a list of guidelines for selecting engineering controls (United States Department of Labor, 1991):

1. Designing workstations to accommodate the people who actually work on a given job, not the "average" person or typical worker. Workstations should be easily adjustable and either designed or selected to fit a specific task, so they are comfortable for the workers using them. The workspace should be large enough to allow for the full range of required movements, especially when knives, saws, hooks, and similar tools are used
2. Designing work methods to reduce static, extreme, and awkward postures; repetitive motion; and excessive force. Work method design addresses the content of tasks performed by the workers. It requires analysis of the production system to design or modify tasks to eliminate stressors

3. Designing tools and handles to reduce the risk of cumulative trauma disorders (CTD). Tools should be available in a variety of sizes to achieve a proper fit and reduce ergonomic risk. The appropriate tool should be used to do a specific job. Tools and handles should be selected to eliminate or minimize the following stressors:

- Chronic muscle contraction or steady force
- Extreme or awkward finger, hand, or arm positions
- Repetitive forceful motions
- Tool vibration
- Excessive gripping, pinching, or pressing with the hand and fingers

Conclusion

A knowledge and understanding of ergonomic principles and their applications can provide the foundation for the development of ergonomic interventions, including job analysis and injury prevention programs. The suggestions herein provide therapists with variables to consider in the development and implementation of a job analysis. It is essential to note that the information in this book represents a variety of perspectives and is intended as a guide for ergonomic intervention. Each job is different; it has unique features, functions, and demands. These unique characteristics make the process a challenge for therapists within industry and health care.

References

Armstrong, T.J. (1986). Ergonomics and cumulative trauma disorders. Hand Clinics, 2:553-565.

Bell, N.N. (1991). Oh, my aching back! Business & Health, April:63-68.

Buckle, P., Stubbs, D. (1989). The contribution of ergonomics to the rehabilitation of back pain patients. Journal of the Society of Occupational Medicine, 39:56-60.

Bureau of National Affairs (1988). Back Injuries: Cost, Causes, & Prevention (pp. 75-109). Washington, D.C.: Bureau of National Affairs.

Burrous, N.L. (1988). An industrial response to low-back injuries and their prevention. In M.K. Campbell (Ed.), Topics in Acute Care and Trauma Rehabilitation: Industrial Back Injuries (pp. 78-83). Part I. Rockville, Md.: Aspen.

Grandjean, E. (1988). Fitting the Task to the Man: A Textbook of Occupational Ergonomics, 4th ed. (p. 205). Bristol, Pa.:Taylor & Francis.

Gross, C.M. (1990). Reduce musculoskeletal injuries with corporate ergonomics program. Occupational Health and Safety, January: 28-33.

Haag, A. (1992). Ergonomic standards, guidelines, and strategies for prevention of back injury. Occupational Medicine, 7:155-165.

Industry Safety Tips from the Alliance: Saving Lives, Boosting Production, Cutting Insurance Costs (1985). Journal of American Insurance, (fourth quarter):11-14.

Isernhagen, S.J. (1988). Work Injury: Management and Prevention (pp. 19-22). Rockville, Md.: Aspen.

Jackson, L.C. (1991). Ergonomics and the occupational health nurse: Instituting a workplace program. AAOHN Journal, 39:119-127.

Joyce, M. (1988). Ergonomics offers solutions to numerous health complaints. Occupational Health and Safety, 58:65-66.

Kazutaka, K. (1989). Training in practical ergonomics improvements. Journal of Human Ergology, 18:147-150.

Lutz, G., Hansford, T. (1987). Cumulative trauma disorder controls: The ergonomics program at Ethicon, Inc. Journal of Hand Surgery, 12A:863-869.

Lutz, G., Hansford, T. (1991). Ethicon, Inc: A Success Story. Ergonomics 1:5-6.

MacLeod, D., Jacobs, P., Larson, N. (1990). The Ergonomics Manual. Minneapolis, Minn.:CLMI Ergotech.

McCasland, L.J. (1992). Development of an ergonomic program for the meatpacking industry. AAOHN Journal, 40:138-142.

McReynolds, M.A. (1991). Managing the high cost of back injury. Occupational Health and Safety, 58:62-64.

Moffett, J.A. Klaber, Chase, S.M., Portek, I., Ennis, J.R. (1986). A controlled, prospective study to evaluate the effectiveness of a back school in the relief of chronic low back pain. Spine, 11:120-122.

Moretz, S. (1989). Ergonomics power plant's safety upsurge. Occupational Hazards, March:27-29.

Pheasant, S. (1991). Ergonomics, Work and Health. Gaithersburg, Md.: Aspen.

Putz-Anderson, V. (Ed.) (1991). Cumulative Trauma Disorders: A Manual for Musculoskeletal Diseases of the Upper Limbs. New York: Taylor & Francis.

Schumacher, A. (1990). Getting a back injury program back on track. Safety & Health, November:44-47.

Schwartz, R.K. (1990). Preventing the incurable: Proactive risk management. Work, 1:12-26.

Snook, S.H. (1978). The design of manual handling tasks. Ergonomics, 21:963-986.

Snook, S.H. (1988). Approaches to the control of back pain in industry: Job placement and education/training. Occupational Medicine, 3:45-59.

Stultz, M.R. (1990). Low back injury prevention via training: An analysis of program components and their effectiveness. Occupational Safety and Health Engineering, 13:1-22.

Travers, P.H. (1992). Implementing ergonomic strategies in the workplace: An occupational health nursing perspective. AAOHN Journal, 40:129-137.

United States Department of Labor. Dictionary of Occupational Titles. Washington, D.C.: United States Department of Labor.

United States Department of Labor Occupational Safety and Health Administration (1991). Ergonomics Program Management Guidelines for Meatpacking Plants. Washington, D.C.: U.S. Government Printing Office.

Versloot, J.M., Rozeman, A., van Son, A.M., Van Akkerveeken, P.F. (1992). The cost effectiveness of a back school program in industry: A longitudinal controlled field study. Spine, 17:22-27.

CHAPTER 12

Marketing Ergonomic Consultation

Karen Jacobs

ABSTRACT

Marketing is an important aspect of the delivery of services. This chapter provides an overview of marketing with a focus on ergonomic consultation. A case study is provided to illustrate the application of marketing strategies in the development of a new product.

Question: What do a microwave oven and ergonomic consultation have in common?
Answer: They are both products that have been developed in response to consumers' needs.

The microwave oven was invented to meet the needs of two-career couples who had little time to spend on food preparation. Ergonomic consultation in occupational and physical therapy evolved to meet the need to curtail rising health care and worker compensation costs brought about by an increased number of industrial injuries and the need to prevent injuries in the workplace.

Product development that takes place in response to the changing needs and wants of the public is part of a marketing approach. Since the early 1980s marketing has become more common in health care. In fact, marketing has become necessary to survive in a competitive marketplace. However, traditionally, therapists developed their products based on what they believed the customer wanted relative to their own plans. Marketing reverses this process.

Marketing is an important aspect of the delivery of services in today's changing health care environment, and it is critical that all therapists understand marketing. Therapists need to learn how to use the techniques of marketing just as they needed to go to school to learn how to use the tools and techniques of their profession. Limited exposure to marketing, if any, is provided in the academic curriculum of occupational and physical therapists. Therefore, it is highly recommended that therapists acquire this marketing knowledge by attending workshops, taking continuing education courses, or acquiring degrees in business. In general, therapists need to become more business savvy.

A Definition of Marketing

Marketing is a misunderstood term. It is most often used synonymously with public relations, selling, fund-raising, strategic planning, or development. According to Kotler (1975, p. 5)

> Marketing is the analysis, planning, implementation and control of carefully formulated programs designed to bring about voluntary exchanges of values with target markets for the purpose of achieving organizational objectives. It relies heavily on designing the organization's offering in terms of the target market's needs and desires, and on using effective pricing, communication, and distribution to inform, motivate and service the markets. . . .

Paramount in this definition are needs and desires. Something that is perceived as lacking by the market (an individual or group of individuals) reflects a need; a desire is a want or personal preference. Through market research, the market is analyzed to determine whether it reflects an absence of a good or service or whether it prefers something in a different shape, form, time, or location. According to Kiernan et al (1989, p. 50)

> Once the need or want is established, the potential buyer must view the good or service being offered as satisfying a need or want better than any other available good or service. It is the packaging and support of a good or service that assure an ongoing relationship with the customer both for purposes of repurchase and for influencing initial purchases by other potential buyers.

Marketing should be viewed as a dynamic activity that includes the successful analysis of a need, the design of a good or service to meet the need, the uniting of that good or service with a potential user, and the use of a good or service by the customer. In the ideal situation, a marketing approach is used before a product is developed. This has not always been the case. In particular, many industrial rehabilitation programs (eg, work hardening) that may have begun with a selling perspective are now faced with the risk of having been developed as products for which there is no longer a need particularly at their cost or present locations (Jacobs, 1991).

A Marketing Approach

There are four components to a marketing approach: (1) analyzing market opportunities; (2) researching and selecting target markets and market segments; (3) developing marketing strategies; and (4) executing and evaluating the marketing plan.

Analyzing Market Opportunities

The first step in a marketing approach is the analysis of various elements in the marketplace. The market itself needs to be defined and may be selected simply on the basis of geographic territory. The market is all actual or potential buyers of a product, service, or idea. In the case of ergonomic consultation, some markets are industry, occupational health or rehabilitation nurses, insurance companies, safety officers, lawyers, injured workers, and allied health professionals. Identifying attractive target markets includes the analysis of marketing opportunities. This analysis consists of a self-audit, consumer analysis, competition analysis, and environmental assessment (Jacobs, 1989).

Self-audit

A self-audit assesses the strengths and weaknesses of, opportunities for, and threats to (SWOT analysis) the individual therapist, service, or organization. Factors to be assessed might include the following:

1. The reputation of the organization in the community. For example, does the organization or individual therapist have a good reputation in the community?
2. The therapists' qualifications. For example, do the therapists have master's degrees or specialized training in ergonomics or human factors or biomechanics? Are any of the therapists certified as professional ergonomists or eligible for certification? (see Chapter 13)
3. Finances. For example, is state-of-the-art equipment available to perform job site analysis, or can it be purchased if needed? Is the individual or company eligible to apply for grant funding, for example, to develop "Train the Trainer" workshops at a designated work site?

This self-audit assists in understanding how well or poorly prepared an individual or business is to meet the demands of the marketplace. Ascertaining what an individual or business does well and maintaining that product or service at an optimal level is a critical aspect of marketing.

Consumer analysis

The potential consumers must be identified for the provider to understand their needs and wants for the product. Examples of consumers who might need or use ergonomic consultation are business and industry, occupational health or rehabilitation nurses, insurance companies, architects, attorneys, safety officers, injured workers, and allied health professionals.

Competition analysis

Identifying other providers of similar services gives an overview of the kinds of services being offered in a particular locale. Analyzing these services reduces the potential for overlap and helps identify areas that are not being served. Opportunities for collaboration or joint ventures may surface during the competition analysis.

Environmental assessment

An environmental assessment predicts the role present and future demographics, political and regulatory systems, cultural and economic environments, psychographics, and technology may have on services. The following provide environmental factors that have an impact on ergonomics: demographics, political and regulatory agencies, and economic and financial factors.

Demographics. Through economic necessity or preference, many older Americans remain in or reenter the work force after the traditional age of retirement. In the United States, 11% of the population, or 24 million people, have reached or passed the age of 65 years. By 2034, this percentage is expected to increase to 18%. By the year 2050, 25% of the United States population will be in this age group; many will be even older. To keep this working population active, occupational and physical therapists must become familiar with the aging process and learn to recognize the special needs of older workers. By becoming familiar with the physiologic effects of aging, therapists will be able to develop treatment plans and prevention strategies that use ergonomic principles (Coy & Davenport, 1991).

Political and Regulatory Agencies. The Occupational Safety and Health Administration (OSHA) has published guidelines for the meat-packing industry called "Ergonomic Program Management Guidelines for Meatpacking Plants" (OSHA, 1991). Although these guidelines are specific to meat-packing, they are useful for an overall ergonomic program for most work sites. OSHA is in the process of developing "Ergonomic Program Management Guidelines for General Industry." These standards will increase the need for qualified consultants to assist industry in compliance. In addition, the Department of Labor has released the document "Ergonomics and the Americans with Disabilities Act," which states that people who suffer from ergonomic disorders are covered by the Americans with Disabilities Act (ADA) if the physical or mental impairment substantially limits the ability to perform the essential functions of the job (cited in Smith, 1993, p. 8).

On a state level, there is movement toward the establishment of guidelines or standards for the use of video display terminals (VDTs). These standards will be established by January 1, 1995, in California. In New York City, city employees receive frequent breaks, regular eye examinations, ergonomically designed furniture, and training to reduce disorders associated with VDT use (Bloswick, 1993). Therapists interested in consulting in industry must develop an understanding of these guidelines and keep current with new standards.

Economic and Financial Factors. By the 21st century, 50% of the work force will suffer some type of occupational disorder. The cost to society will be billions of dollars each year (Sutherland & Counihan, 1990). For example, low-back pain accounts for millions of days lost from work and billions of dollars of lost productivity and worker compensation claims. Clearly, injury prevention at the work site and health promotion are better alternatives to injury management (Jacobs, 1992). The economic and financial benefits of injury prevention programs include less lost work time, increased safety and productivity, reduced errors, improved quality of service, and better employee relations (Sehnal & Christopher, 1993). Good ergonomics can mean good economics.

Researching and Selecting Target Markets

Once the marketing opportunities have been analyzed, the needs of the market can be determined through research, which might include observation, survey, or even experimentation to test hypotheses. After research is completed, the market is divided into target markets, that is, groups of consumers with similar needs, wants, or interests. The groups are further segmented into distinct groups of consumers who might require separate products and promotions. For example, industry can be segmented into types of businesses, or service industries and manufacturing industries. Service industry can be further segmented into organizations within a certain geographic area. Targeting a market is the act of evaluating and selecting one or more of the markets to enter.

Developing Marketing Strategies

The marketing approach continues by developing a marketing mix to meet the needs, wants, or interests of this well-defined target market. It is what can be done to influence the demand for a product or service. A marketing mix consists of the four Ps: product, price, place, and promotion.

Product

The product is a marketing variable that needs to be designed for the specific target market. For example, for ergonomic consultation to a hospital, the products or product line might include job-site analysis; an audit for compliance with Titles II and III of the ADA; recommending intervention for injured workers, such as splinting, or a designing or redesigning of the workstation (eg, changing the height of a table, counter, or chair); and implementing preventive programs, such as health promotion on the work site, including stress management or physical exercise.

Place

Where the product or service is provided is the place component of the marketing mix. Ergonomic consultation is usually provided at the work site; however, on occasion, therapists provide consultation in their own offices or provide expert testimony in a court of law.

Price

The price or fee schedule for services should be based on cost, competitive factors, geographic area, and what the consumer is willing to pay. The four important methods for establishing a fee schedule are unit value system; cost-plus or overhead; local survey, or usual and customary fee; and state code. Whatever method is selected, it is important for the price to be commensurate with perceived value.

Promotion

Promotion is the vehicle of communicating information to the consumer about the merits, place, and price of the product. According to Folts et al (1993, p. 13)

> Work programs do not sell services; rather, they sell the benefits of those services. Clients do not want therapeutic modalities, exercises, or purposeful activities. Instead, clients desire the benefits treatment provides, such as pain reduction and the ability to return to work.

Instruments of promotion are advertising, sales promotion, publicity, and personal selling.

Advertising.   Advertising involves the use of a paid message presented in a recognized medium by an identified sponsor with the purpose to inform, persuade, and remind. Some advertising vehicles include brochures, direct mail, or printed advertisement in the client company's monthly newsletter.

Sales Promotion. Sales promotion is the use of a wide variety of short-term incentives to encourage purchase of the product. This approach is optimized when used in conjunction with advertising. For example, at an open house for an industrial rehabilitation program, a successful sales promotion to increase new referrals is a business-card drawing for a free ergonomic job-site analysis (Jacobs, 1994, p. 40).

Publicity. Publicity is underused in relation to the real contribution it can make (Kotler, 1983). Publicity is free promotion. Despite this positive feature, one has little control over placement, and thus it becomes difficult to aim the message at target markets. An example of the use of publicity to promote ergonomic consultation is the use of radio public service announcements on topics such as stress management in the workplace or preventing cumulative trauma disorders (CTD).

Personal Selling. Personal selling is the most effective form of promotion. It is face-to-face communication between the therapist and the consumer. Some examples of personal selling are making presentations at meetings, providing continuing education workshops, or lecturing to professional organizations. In addition, word-of-mouth recommendations by past recipients of ergonomic consultation are a powerful sales tool.

Executing and Evaluating the Marketing Plan

Once the target market has been selected and the marketing mix developed, the marketing plan is implemented. Because marketing is a dynamic activity, the plan requires continual evaluation of its effectiveness. A specific time frame, such as a 12-month period, should be delineated to measure whether objectives and goals are being met. The marketing plan should be flexible so that changes can be made as new opportunities and problems arise.

Conclusion

The use of a marketing approach allows therapists to take a proactive approach in the health care environment and be ready to meet the changing needs and wants of the marketplace.
    According to Schwartz (1991, p.365)

> Occupational therapy is strategically placed to assume a leadership role in work place injury prevention. . . . Prevention services offered by occupational therapists both minimize the incidence and severity of disability, for a far lower

cost than occupational health physicians and other primary care providers have traditionally charged.

Case Study

This case study demonstrates the use of marketing before the expansion of services.

A well-established, free-standing industrial rehabilitation center planned to begin including ergonomic consultation in its line of services. The director of the center decided to perform a market analysis to ascertain the feasibility of expanding the product line. The first step was to identify attractive target markets. In identifying these markets, the director performed an analysis of marketing opportunities—a self audit, a consumer analysis, a competitive analysis, and an environmental assessment.

Self-audit

A SWOT analysis was performed to ascertain the strengths and weaknesses of, opportunities for, and threats to the center.

Strengths

- Three occupational and physical therapists with master's degrees. Two of these therapists were Certified Professional Ergonomists (CPEs).
- An excellent reputation in the community
- A location in an area with a high concentration of plastics and paper manufacturers

Weakness

- Limited financial resources for the purchase of equipment needed for job-site analysis

Opportunities

- The medical director of the center had been appointed medical director of a local plastics-manufacturing company
- The center was eligible to apply for state funding provided by the Department of Industrial Accidents to develop a proposal for ergonomic training for companies with workers at risk for CTD

Threats

- Two local physical therapists in private practice were expanding services to include ergonomic consultation

Consumer Analysis

The consumer analysis revealed the following markets as potential users of ergonomic consultation:

- Local industry, in particular manufacturers whose employees performed repetitive upper-extremity tasks and material handling, eg, paper manufacturers
- Employees who worked extensively at VDTs, such as insurance agency personnel

Competitive Analysis

A competitive analysis revealed two competitors within a 30-mile radius of the center. These competitors had been identified in the self-audit under the "threat" category.

Environmental Assessment

An environmental assessment indicated that the center was located in a industrial community with an aging work force. One manufacturer of plastics noted that over the last 2 years an increasing number of workers sustained CTD. Concurrently, the number of lost work days per 100 workers increased steadily.

Market Segmentation

Over a 2-week period the market analysis was completed, and a market segmentation was proposed. That is, the potential consumers of ergonomic consultation were divided into distinct groups. For example, physicians were segmented into orthopedic surgeons, occupational health practitioners, and neurologists. This market was further defined by the selection of only occupational health physicians as the proposed primary referral source for ergonomic consultation. Market segmentation was also performed for industrial sites.

Developing marketing strategies specific to each target market was the next step in the analysis. That is, the optimal marketing mix of product, place, price, and promotion had to be devised. One of the target markets was a local plastics manufacturer. The center's product line for this manufacturer included baseline ergonomic screening surveys, job-site analyses, customized education and training programs, work-site modifications, and product design and evaluation (see Chapter 6 for more information on product design and evaluation). Ergonomic consultation would be provided at the work site, and the price of services would be based on cost-plus in consideration with what the competition was charging.

Promotion was aimed at the plastics industry. It was proposed that the most effective mechanism was personal selling. That is, one of the therapists would contact the director of human resources of the plastics manufacturer and arrange for an appointment to promote ergonomic consultation. It also was proposed that a brochure be developed to delineate the center's expanded product line of ergonomic consultation. A time line was proposed to measure whether the strategies achieved the desired result of obtaining a contract for ergonomic consultation.

When the market analysis was completed, it appeared feasible to expand the center's product line to include ergonomic consultation on a trial basis (12 months). The director would evaluate the strategies after 6 months and again at the end of the year to determine if the goals and objectives were being met.

References

Bloswick, D. (1993). Developing ergonomics programs in industry: A practical guide. Salt Lake City: University of Utah.

Coy, J., Davenport, M. (1991). Age changes in the older adult worker: Implications for injury prevention. Work, 2:38-46.

Folts, D., Jeremko, J., Houk, D. (1993). Marketing's role in work programs. Work, 3:13-18.

Jacobs, K. (1989). Work hardening in the health care system. In L. Ogden-Niemeyer, K. Jacobs (Eds.), Work Hardening: State of the Art (pp. 111-126). Thorofare: Slack.

Jacobs K. (1991). A marketing approach to work practice. Work Programs Special Interest Section Newsletter, 5:3-4.

Jacobs, K. (1992). From the Editor. Work, 2:1.

Jacobs, K. (1994). Marketing occupational therapy services. In Jacobs K., Logigian M. (Eds.). Functions of a Manager in Occupational Therapy (pp. 33-49). Thorofare: Slack.

Kiernan, W., Carter, A., Bronstein, E. (1989). Marketing and marketing management in rehabilitation. In W. Kiernan, R. Schalock (Eds.), Economics, Industry, and Disability (pp. 49-56). Baltimore: Brookes.

Kotler, P. (1975). Marketing for non profit organizations. Englewood Cliffs: Prentice-Hall.

Kotler, P. (1983). Principles of Marketing: Instructor's Manual with Cases. Englewood Cliffs: Prentice-Hall.

Schwartz, R. (1991). Prevention. In Jacobs, K. (Ed.), Occupational Therapy: Work Related Programs and Assessments (pp. 365-381). Boston: Little, Brown.

Sehnal, J., Christopher, R. (1993). Developing and marketing an ergonomics program in a corporate office environment. Work, 3:22-30.

Smith, M. (1993). Ergonomic update: Legislative, judicial, and other happenings. Preventing Injury, 2:8-9.

Sutherland, R., Counihan, W. (1990). Functional restoration for the back-injured worker: A sports medicine approach. Occupational Therapy Practice, 1:11-26.
U.S. Department of Labor Occupational Health and Safety Administration [OSHA] (1991). Ergonomic program management guidelines for meatpacking plants.

CHAPTER 13

Certification in Ergonomics

Karen Jacobs

ABSTRACT

The establishment of a credentialing process in ergonomics would provide some type of quality control in
this arena. The Board for Certification in Professional
Ergonomics (BCPE) and two other groups are described
in this brief overview.

For many years, the Human Factors Society (HFS) has been concerned about
establishing some type of quality control or credentialing of ergonomists.
However, this issue was tabled in 1987. The efforts were renewed in October
of 1990 with the formation of an independent certification and professional
development organization called the Board for Certification in Professional
Ergonomics (BCPE). Two other groups (Health Rehabilitation Ergonomists
and the Medical Ergonomics Society), which are composed primarily of
health care professionals, have been developing other types of certifications
(Rice, 1994b). At present, only the BCPE certification is in place.

Certifications

Criteria for Certification Developed by the BCPE

BCPE has prepared a monograph entitled, "Information on Certification
Policies, Practices & Procedures" (2nd edition, August 1994) that "is intended
to acquaint people aspiring to the designation of Certified Professional

Ergonomist (CPE) or Certified Human Factors Professional (CHFP) with the policies, practices and procedures established by the Board of Certification in Professional Ergonomics" (p. iii). To eliminate the loss of a great deal of time and effort, therapists interested in certification should read this monograph thoroughly prior to obtaining an application.

The certification process for BCPE has two phases. The minimum criteria for both phases are listed below with the exception that those who qualified under Phase I, which ended December 31, 1993, were able to waive the written examination requirement.

1. a master's degree in ergonomics or human factors, or an equivalent educational background in the life sciences, engineering sciences, *and* behavioral sciences to comprise a professional level of ergonomics education, and
2. four (4) years of full-time professional practice as an ergonomist practitioner with emphasis on design involvement (derived from ergonomic analysis and/or ergonomic testing/evaluation), and
3. documentation of education, employment history, and ergonomic project involvement by means of the BCPE "Application for Certification," and
4. a passing score of the BCPE written examination (waived in Phase I) and
5. payment of all fees levied by the BCPE for processing and maintenance of certification, in accordance with the following schedule (BCPE, 1994 p. 7):

Application Fee: U.S. $10.00
Processing and Examination Fee: U.S. $190.00
Annual Certification Maintenance Fee: U.S. $75.00

A person meeting the minimum requirements can initiate the certification process by requesting an application by sending a $10.00 check to BCPE, P.O. Box 2811, Bellingham, WA 98227-2811; (206) 671-7601; (206) 671-7681 (FAX).

Once the application has been completed, it is evaluated by the review panel and recommendations are made to the board whether or not the applicant qualifies to take the written examination.

Phase I

According to Mr. Dieter W. Jahns, M.C., CPE, executive director of BCPE, there were 701 applicants under Phase I. As of October 5, 1994, 524 applicants were certified: 89 were in some process of evaluation, and 88 had been deferred to the examination. Of the 524 applicants who were certified, four were occupational therapists and three were physical therapists (Lt. Colonel Valerie Rice, Ph.D., OTR/L, CPE, personal communication, July 9, 1994,

Boston, Mass.) Since therapists are still in some process of evaluation, I would anticipate that these numbers will change.

Phase II

Under the ongoing Phase II, applicants continue to apply to sit for the exam (Mr. Dieter W. Jahns, M.S., CPE, executive director of BCPE, personal communication, October 5, 1994).

Written Examination

A rigorous full-day examination is scheduled each spring and fall. It is anticipated that the examination will be offered as an adjunct to the meetings of ergonomics related professional societies and associations (BCPE, 1994, p. 8.)

The examination has three sections and "is designed and constructed to examine both fundamental knowledge in ergonomics (Test Section I: 2.0 hours) by means of multiple-choice items and application skills by means of written answers to questions spanning the practices and principles appropriately applied in a setting of ergonomists' involvement with systems analysis, ergonomic design, and systems/human performance evaluation (Test Section II: 2.5 hours, and Test Section III: 2.5 hours)" (BCPE, 1994, pp. 9-10.)

As cited in BCPE's "Information on Certification Policies, Practices & Procedures," the following are some sample questions from each section:

Section I: Fundamental Knowledge (Sample Question)

The boundaries of a system are:

a. obvious and cannot be changed.
b. defined such that the system performs an identifiable function.
c. set so that everything that affects the system is inside the boundary.
d. constantly changing and cannot be defined.

Section II: Principles, Methods, and Techniques (Sample Question)

List the four primary functions of a human-machine system.

Section III: Ergonomic Problem Solving

To assess the applicant's ergonomic problem-solving capabilities, Section III poses several realistic scenarios requiring professional involvement.

Sample Problem Scenario and Related Questions: A support group for severely handicapped people has decided to build apartments in which to house them. The goal is to allow them to function in the apartments as independently as possible. Because design guidelines for the nonhandicapped do not apply, the group hires you to develop and test an ergonomic design that will satisfy the need. List and describe the ergonomic problems presumed in the scenario or the steps you would take to define the ergonomic problems.

Future Considerations

Since, "the dynamics of technological and societal change make ergonomics a rapidly evolving career field . . . professional-practice-standards developed by the BCPE is a continuous improvement process. Issues such as 'speciality-practice areas' within ergonomics based on diverse educational backgrounds; multi-level certifications conforming to ergonomics skill levels of practitioners; CEU [Continuing Education Units] requirements for certification (and skill/knowledge) maintenance; and certificate revocation criteria are being actively explored" (BCPE, 1994, p. iii).

Health/Rehabilitation Ergonomists

The Ergonomic Rehabilitation Research Society (ERRS), dedicated to the scientific analysis of the prevention of disability and restoration of function, acted as the catalyst to bring together a group of 15 health care practitioners in July 1993 to discuss ergonomics as it applies to them (Rice, 1994b, p. 71-72). These health care practitioners, referred to as NACHRE, or the National Interdisciplinary Committee on Health and Rehabilitation Ergonomics, provided expertise "in the development of guidelines for the involvement of health care professionals in the practice of ergonomics and industrial rehabilitation" (Hart et al, 1993, p. 71-72). During this time, a dialogue was established with the BCPE to explore possible certification under the board. A proposal was sent to the BCPE and feedback was provided that it was too broad and that it would be better to narrow the focus to include rehabilitation ergonomic professionals doing ergonomics for injured workers or for healthy workers who might be in high risk jobs. In August 1994, founders of ERRS, Dr. Leonard Matheson, Ph.D., Susan J. Isernhagen, PT, and Dr. Dennis L. Hart, Ph.D., PT, met in Washington to narrow the scope of the rehabilitation ergonomist. This narrowed scope has been documented and was sent to members of NACHRE for their approval. By early 1995 a revised proposal is scheduled to be submitted to BCPE.

For more information contact: Dr. Leonard Matheson, Ph.D., ERIC, Inc., 600 South Grand, Santa Ana, CA 92705, (714) 836-1224; (714) 836-0227 (fax).

Medical Ergonomist

The Medical Ergonomics Society (MES) proposes a certification for qualified physicians as medical ergonomists. According to Rice (1994a, p. 212), "The emphasis of the role of the Medical Ergonomist is on health care delivery using a systems approach." The proposal includes a terminal degree, professional licensure, a baseline level of work experience, and a submission of work products. The MES has contacted the BCPE regarding certification.

Discussion

The impact of certification by these groups on the practice of ergonomics is open to question. The positive scenario might be better control of the quality of services and services that are more cost-effective than in the past. An alternative scenario might be an increased misunderstanding on the part of consumers and third-party reimbursers about the areas of service that are the domain of Certified Professional Ergonomists or Certified Human Factors Professionals as opposed to health ergonomists as opposed to medical ergonomists as opposed to health care professionals with no certification and about who is best qualified to provide these services. Many other alternative scenarios may evolve. Only time will tell. The use of marketing strategies may assist qualified therapists to stay competitive in the health care system and to maintain their market share in ergonomic consultation. The reader is advised to keep abreast of certification through updates in the quarterly journal, *WORK: A Journal of Prevention, Assessment & Rehabilitation.*

References

BCPE, (1994). Information on Certification Policies, Practices & Procedures, 2nd ed. Bellingham, Wash.: BCPE.

Hart, D., Isernhagen, S., Matheson, L., (1993). Refining the practice of ergonomics, Work 3 (3): 69-72.

Rice, V. (1994a). Certification in ergonomics: An update and commentary. Work, 4(1):211-213.

Rice, V. (1994b). Ergonomics certification update. Work, 4(1):71-72.

Appendixes

Appendix 1

WORK SITE JOB ANALYSIS AND DESIGN CONSIDERATIONS

1. Job Organization /Structure
   A. Hours/Shift
   B. Breaks
   C. Rest periods
   D. Job rotation
   E. Piece work
   F. Job-rate quotas
   G. Production incentives
   H. Work pace
   I. Work schedule

2. Tools and Equipment
   A. Weight and size
   B. Mechanical aids for heavy tools and equipment
   C. Balancers
   D. Sharpness
   E. Location
   F. Condition
   G. Temperature
   H. Power vs. manual
   I. Grasping surface, friction, and slip resistance
   J. Glove use and fit
   K. Ability to slide vs. lifting
   L. Torque
   M. Force requirements
   N. Handles
      1. Size and shape
      2. Thickness/diameter
      3. Grip or pinch design
      4. Serrations
      5. Friction with hand
      6. Length
      7. Surface material
      8. Compressibility (wood, metal, rubber)
      9. Heat or electrical conductivity
      10. Sharp edges

11. Hand-tool position/posture
12. Ability to use in both hands
13. Dampening-material coating to minimize vibration

O. Padding, bolsters, and cushions
P. Curved vs. sharp edges and corners of tools and equipment
Q. Use of tools vs. hands for pounding
R. Foot pedal use, location, position, and number

3. Manual Materials Handling
    A. Force and weight of load
    B. Location of load in relation to the worker
        1. Horizontal distance
        2. Vertical distance
        3. Amount of twisting required to handle material
        4. Storage position for accessibility
    C. Size of load/container
    D. Load stability
    E. Location of coupling/handles/cutouts
    F. Mechanical aid availability (carts, hoists, scissoring pallets/tables, two-wheelers)
    G. Automation availability
    H. Lifting frequency
    I. Working surface (texture, level, spills)
    J. Worker availability for two-person lifts
    K. Workplace layout and design
        1. Location/height of shelving, tables, and benches in order to position loads at easily accessible levels
        2. Presence of barriers/obstacles in work area
        3. Movement quality, symmetry, and balance during worktime
        4. Posture during work time/cycle
    L. Environmental factors
        1. Lighting/illumination
        2. Vibration
        3. Temperature/humidity
        4. Noise level
        5. Air quality/circulation
    M. Age and gender
    N. NIOSH lifting equation

4. Controls and Display Presentation
    A. Type of information
    B. Ease of reach for frequently used controls
    C. Feedback to indicate that control has been activated (tactile, auditory, visual)

D. Information complexity (easy to read and identify)
E. Size, shape, and color for control emphasis
F. Placement of guards to prevent accidental activation
G. Viewing distance, angle, and lighting

5. Seated Work
    A. Chair
        1. Height adjustability
        2. Seat pan width and depth
        3. Backrest/lumbar support and adjustability
        4. Armrests
        5. Footrests/support
        6. Caster base
        7. Maneuverability
        8. Ease of adjustment operation
        9. Size, appearance, overall comfort
        10. Type of work performed during chair use
    B. Ease of job in seated position
    C. Location of objects to be lifted
    D. Location of objects to be handled
    E. Height of work surface
    F. Ability to alternate sitting and standing
    G. Dynamic vs. static nature of work
    H. Posture
    I. Stretch breaks

6. Standing Work
    A. Standing surface
    B. Antifatigue mates
    C. Cushion-soled shoes/inserts
    D. Height of work surface
    E. Location of objects/equipment
    F. Rails, bars, stools for footrest
    G. Ability to alternate standing and sitting
    H. Sit-stand–type chairs
    I. Dynamic vs. static nature of work
    J. Posture
    K. Stretch breaks

7. Psychosocial Environment
    A. Task/job complexity
    B. Monotony and repetition
    C. Peer/social support
    D. Worker autonomy

   E.   Accuracy requirements
   F.   Excessive job task speed or load
   G.   Sensory deprivation and isolation

Appendix 2

AMERICANS WITH DISABILITIES ACT WORK SITE ASSESSMENT

Company: Areas Evaluated:
_____

Address: Telephone:
_____

Job Title: Primary Function of Company:
_____

Contact Person:
_____

Reason for Referral:
_____

Date: Evaluated by:
_____

Method of Evaluation:

_____ Observation of worker

_____ Simulation of job by worker

_____ Discussion of job with (identity)

_____ Review of company job description

_____ Review of *Dictionary of Occupational Titles* (DOT)
_____

Signature of Company Representative:

_____

Terms:

Sedentary Work: lift 10 lb maximum; occasionally carry small objects
Light Work: lift 20 lb maximum; frequently lift or carry up to 10 lb
Medium Work: lift 20 lb maximum; frequently lift or carry up to 25 lb
Heavy Work: lift 100 lb maximum; frequently lift or carry up to 50 lb
Very Heavy Work: lift in excess of 100 lb; frequently lift or carry 50 lb

In terms of an 8-hour workday: Constantly   67% to 100%
                                  Frequently   34% to 66%
                                  Occasionally   1% to 33%
_____

Brief Description of Job:

_____

Functional Body Positions

What is the maximal requirement of sitting necessary for the job?
_____ constantly _____ frequently _____ occasionally _____never
_____ essential   _____ marginal

What is the worker actually doing while sitting?

What is the maximal requirement of standing necessary for the job?
_____ constantly _____ frequently _____ occasionally _____never
_____ essential   _____ marginal

What is the worker actually doing while standing?

What is the maximal requirement of walking necessary for the job?
_____ constantly _____ frequently _____ occasionally _____never
_____ essential   _____ marginal

What is the worker actually doing while walking?

What is the maximal requirement of climbing necessary for the job?
_____ constantly _____ frequently _____ occasionally _____never
_____ essential   _____ marginal

What is the worker actually doing while climbing?

What is the maximal requirement of balancing necessary for the job?
_____ constantly _____ frequently _____ occasionally _____never
_____ essential   _____ marginal

What is the worker actually doing while balancing?

What is the maximal requirement of stooping necessary for the job?
_____ constantly _____ frequently _____ occasionally _____never
_____ essential   _____ marginal

What is the worker actually doing while stooping?

What is the maximal requirement of kneeling necessary for the job?
_____ constantly _____ frequently _____ occasionally _____never
_____ essential   _____ marginal

What is the worker actually doing while kneeling?

What is the maximal requirement of crouching necessary for the job?
_____ constantly _____ frequently _____ occasionally _____never
_____ essential   _____ marginal

What is the worker actually doing while crouching?

_____

What is the maximal requirement of crawling necessary for the job?
_____ constantly _____ frequently _____ occasionally ____never
_____ essential   _____ marginal

_____

What is the worker actually doing while crawling?

_____

What is the maximal requirement of pulling necessary for the job?
_____ constantly _____ frequently _____ occasionally ____never
_____ essential   _____ marginal

_____

What is the worker actually doing while pulling?

_____

What is the maximal requirement of pushing necessary for the job?
_____ constantly _____ frequently _____ occasionally ____never
_____ essential   _____ marginal

_____

What is the worker actually doing while pushing?

_____

What is the maximal requirement of fingering necessary for the job?
_____ constantly _____ frequently _____ occasionally ____never
_____ essential   _____ marginal

_____

What is the worker actually doing while fingering?

_____

What is the maximal requirement of feeling necessary for the job?
_____ constantly _____ frequently _____ occasionally ____never
_____ essential   _____ marginal

_____

What is the worker actually doing while feeling?

_____

What is the maximal requirement of reaching at shoulder height or overhead necessary for the job?
_____ constantly _____ frequently _____ occasionally ____never
_____ essential   _____ marginal

_____

What is the worker actually doing while reaching at shoulder height or overhead? (Include reaching distance.)

_____

What is the maximal requirement of reaching below shoulder height for the job?
_____ constantly _____ frequently _____ occasionally ____never
_____ essential   _____ marginal

_____

What is the worker actually doing while reaching below shoulder height? (Include reaching distance.)

_____

Environmental Conditions

What is the maximal requirement for inside work necessary to perform the job?
_____ constantly _____ frequently _____ occasionally _____never
_____ essential _____ marginal

What is the worker actually doing when performing inside work?

What is the maximal requirement for outside work necessary for the job?
_____ constantly _____ frequently _____ occasionally _____never
_____ essential _____ marginal

What is the worker actually doing when performing outside work?

Is the worker exposed to cold work temperatures while performing the job?
_____ constantly _____ frequently _____ occasionally _____never
_____ essential _____ marginal

What is the worker actually doing when working in cold temperatures?

Is the worker exposed to hot work temperatures while performing the job?
_____ constantly _____ frequently _____ occasionally _____never
_____ essential _____ marginal

What is the worker actually doing when working in hot temperatures?

Is the worker exposed to wet or humid conditions while performing the job?
_____ constantly _____ frequently _____ occasionally _____never
_____ essential _____ marginal

What is the worker actually doing when performing work in wet or humid conditions?

Is the worker exposed to noise or vibration (circle whichever applies or both) while performing the job?
_____ constantly _____ frequently _____ occasionally _____never
_____ essential _____ marginal

What is the worker actually doing when performing work that exposes him or her to noise or vibration?

Is the worker exposed to hazardous work while performing the job?
_____ constantly _____ frequently _____ occasionally _____never
_____ essential _____ marginal

What is the worker actually doing when performing hazardous work?

Is the worker exposed to fumes, odors, dust, or toxic conditions while performing the job?
_____ constantly _____ frequently _____ occasionally ____never
_____ essential   _____ marginal

What is the worker actually doing when exposed to fumes, odors, dust, or toxic conditions?

Is the worker exposed to poor ventilation when performing the job?
_____ constantly _____ frequently _____ occasionally ____never
_____ essential   _____ marginal

What is the worker actually doing when exposed to poor ventilation?

Intellectual and Credential Demands

Is a specific educational degree, certificate, or license required by federal, state, or professional agencies to perform the job?
_____ yes   _____ no
_____ essential _____ marginal

Credentials required:

Is previous experience required for the job?
_____ yes   _____ no
_____ essential _____ marginal

Communication Demands

Is being able to read necessary to perform the job?
_____ yes   _____ no
_____ essential _____ marginal

Nature of reading required:

Is being able to write necessary to perform the job?
_____ yes   _____ no
_____ essential _____ marginal

Nature of writing required:

Is being able to perform mathematical operations necessary for the job?
_____ yes   _____ no
_____ essential _____ marginal

Nature of mathematics required:

Is being able to see necessary to perform the job?
_____ yes   _____ no
_____ essential _____ marginal

Visual skills required:

Is being able to hear necessary to perform the job?
_____ yes   _____ no
_____ essential _____ marginal

Auditory acuity required:

Is being able to speak necessary to perform the job?
_____ yes   _____ no
_____ essential _____ marginal

Command of language required:

Equipment Use

During a work shift, is nonvehicular machinery or equipment used on the job?
_____ yes_____ no

Name & Function	const	freq	occ	never	essential	marginal	yes	no	yes	no

usage — *on the job training?* — *operator license required?*

During a work shift, is nonvehicular machinery or equipment used on the job?
_____ yes_____ no

Name & Function	const	freq	occ	never	essential	marginal	yes	no	yes	no

usage — *on the job training?* — *operator license required?*

Manual Lifting

Describe how objects are handled during a maximal-output day. Include height, weight, shape, frequency of movement, how the object is manipulated, and for what purpose. (Example: 60-lb rectangular boxes [13" × 10" × 5 inches] are lifted from the floor to a table 30 inches high at a rate of one lift per minute. The boxes are lifted to a table to be opened and the contents sorted.)

Task	H Origin	H Dest.	V Origin	V Dest.	F	Asym. Origin	Asym. Dest.	Coupling	Weight

Recommended Weight Limit (RWL)

$$RWL = LC \times HM \times VM \times AM \times CM \times DM \times FM$$

$$RWL = 51 \text{ lb} \times (10 / H) \times (1 - .0075 |V - 30|) \times (.82 + (1.8 / D) \times (1-.0032A) \times (FM \text{ from table}) \times (CM \text{ from table})$$

©1992, D. Aja, K. Jacobs, D. Hermenau.

Source: Aja, D., Jacobs, K., Hermenau, D. (1992). ADA Work Site Assessment.

Appendix 3

Summary Of Factors To Be Analyzed

    I.   Environmental Conditions
   II.   Social Conditions
  III.   Job Tasks
  IV.   Physical Demands
   V.   Cognitive Demands
  VI.   Classification by Strength Requirements
 VII.   Physical Barriers

Employer Name: _____

Address: _____

Client Name: _____

Job Title: _____

Job Location with Building Name or Number: _____

Date of Visit: _____

Vocational Rehabilitation Specialist: _____

Instructions: Check any of the conditions listed in this analysis that are present in the work area.

I. Environmental Conditions

Condition	Definition
1. _____ Inside	Protected from weather conditions, such as factory or office work or long-distance truck driving
2. _____ Outside	No effective protection from the weather, such as postal work or outdoor labor

Condition	*Definition*
3. _____ Extreme Heat	Temperature sufficiently high to cause marked bodily discomfort, such as working next to a hot stove or furnace or near a hot asphalt-spreading machine
4. _____ Extreme Cold	Temperature sufficiently low as to cause marked bodily discomfort, such as working in a cold-storage room
5. _____ Humid or Wet	Atmospheric conditions in which moisture content is sufficiently high to cause marked bodily discomfort such as using a steam garment-presser, contact with water or other liquids
6. _____ Noise _____ (a) _____ (b)	(a) Sound loud enough to distract workers engaged in mental occupations, such as sounds greater than those made by a single typewriter or office machine. (b) Sound loud enough to cause hearing damage, such as noise greater than 85 decibels, which is approximately equal to being in a car in heavy traffic
7. _____ Vibration	Oscillating movement or strain on the body or extremities from repeated motion or shock that may cause harm if endured day after day, such as operating a jackhammer
8. _____ Mechanical Hazards	Danger to fingers or limbs due to feeding or operating power-driven equipment
9. _____ Electrical Hazards	Danger due to possible electrical shock from electric wires, transformers, or uninsulated electrical parts
10. _____ (a) Fire _____ (b) Hot materials _____ (c) Chemical agents	Danger due to possible burns from any of these causes
11. _____ Radiant Energy	Exposure to radiant energy such as x-rays, radioactive material, or ultraviolet light
12. _____ Poor Ventilation	Insufficient or excessive movement of air or exposure to drafts
13. _____ Moving Objects	Exposure to moving equipment and objects in the immediate work area, such as automobiles, cranes, gurneys, and forklifts
14. _____ Sharp Tools	Exposure to tools or materials with sharp edges

Condition	Definition
15. ____ Cluttered or Slippery Floors	Walking surfaces strewn with equipment, tools, electrical wiring, etc, while work is being done and which may involve a risk of tripping or falling; wet, muddy, oily, or highly polished surfaces, which may cause worker to slip or lose footing
16. ____ Elevated Surfaces	Work occurs in places elevated above the ground, such as catwalks, scaffolds, ladders, and roofs
17. ____ Poor Lighting	Unadjustable lighting conditions that place excessive strain on vision during work. Light conditions that are too dim or too bright, causing glare
18. Exposure to: ____ (a) Fumes ____ (b) Odors ____ (c) Dust ____ (d) Mist ____ (e) Gases	Check specific condition if present

II. Social Conditions

Condition	Definition
19. ____ Working with Others	Job duties that require communication and cooperation with other workers, customers, or the public. Includes social skills and ability to tolerate frustration in dealing with others. Workers who have such jobs are sales clerks, supervisors, police
20. ____ Working around Others	Job duties that require the worker to work independently but near other workers, requiring only minimal verbal contact, such as carpenter on construction crew or assembly line worker
21. ____ Working Alone	Job duties that require independent occupational effort and virtually no contact with fellow workers or the public, such as a writer
22. ____ Supervisor	Job duties that require direct supervision of other workers
23. ____ Contact with Violent or Belligerent People	Job duties require contact with people who may behave or speak in an aggressive, hostile, or threatening manner or with people who have a high probability of such behavior. Workers who have such job duties are police officers, bouncers, or psychiatric aides

Condition		*Definition*
24. _____	Working Shifts that *Do Not* Occur between 8:00 a.m. and 5:00 p.m.	Includes split shifts, rotating shifts, and mandatory overtime. *Does not include flex time, positions in* which worker chooses to work earlier or later
25. _____	Protective Equipment	Equipment workers regularly wear to protect themselves while working, including eye protection, canvas or rubber gloves, safety shoes, hard hats, or brightly colored vests

III. Job Tasks

Is It a Critical Job Task? (yes/no)	*Amount of Time in One Workshift*	*Job Tasks*
_____	_____	1. _____
		_____
		_____
		_____
		_____
		_____
		_____
		_____
_____	_____	2. _____
		_____
		_____
		_____
		_____
		_____
		_____
		_____
_____	_____	3. _____
		_____
		_____
		_____
		_____
		_____
		_____
		_____

IV. Physical Demands

Physical Requirements	Hours Required in an 8-hour Day	Minimum Acitivity Requirements at a Time	Distance	Job Activity
Standing				
Sitting				
Walking				
Lifting				
Carrying				
Pushing				
Climbing				
Balancing				
Bending/ Squatting				
Twisting				
Rotation				
Crawling				
Kneeling on				
Reaching above head				
Reaching at waist level				

V. Cognitive Demands

	Yes	No
1. Job requires complete independence of task?	___	___
2. A moderate amount of supervision is provided for this position?	___	___
3. Minimal supervision is offered but is available upon request?		
4. Written directions available to employee outlining the various steps of the job?	___	___

		Yes	No
5.	Verbal instructions are given initially during training but constant cues are not available to employee concerning the job duties?		
6.	The position is very structured?	___	___
7.	The job is unstructured and requires much input from the employee regarding organization, planning, and sequence of task?	___	___
8.	Which of the following skills are required by the job?		
	Short-term memory	___	___
	Long-term memory	___	___
	Organization	___	___
	Planning	___	___
	Sequencing	___	___
	Verbal fluency	___	___
	Reasoning	___	___
	Judgment	___	___
	Problem solving	___	___
	Safety awareness	___	___
	Visual spatial skills	___	___
	Topographic orientation	___	___
	Fine motor dexterity	___	___
	Gross motor coordination	___	___
9.	The work environment is distractible, eg, busy office, much noise, many people coming in and out?	___	___
10.	Employer appears willing to modify job, eg, provide added supervision, structure, directions?	___	___

VI. Classification By Strength Requirements

Degree Of Strength

Sedentary Work: Lifting 10 lb maximum and occasionally lifting or carrying such articles as ledgers or hand tools. Although a sedentary job is defined as one that involves sitting, some walking and standing may be necessary to perform job duties. Example: Worker sits at a desk most of day, takes dictation and transcribes it on a typewriter, and occasionally walks to various departments. Example: Worker sits at a drawing board, walks occasionally, and carries paper, instruments, and books.

Light Work: Lifting 20 lb maximum with frequent lifting or carrying objects up to 10 lb. Even though weight is negligible, a job is in this category when (1) it requires walking or standing to a considerable degree or (2) it requires sitting most of the time but entails pushing or pulling arm and or leg controls. Example: Worker stands and walks behind a counter of a variety store all working day to wrap and bag articles for customers. Example: Worker walks and stands constantly while arranging records in file cabinets and sits occasionally to sort paper. Example: Worker sits most of day and operates an industrial sewing machine.

Medium Work: Lifting 50 lb maximum with frequent lifting or carrying objects that weigh up to 25 lb. Example: Worker assists in lifting patients, pushing gurneys, and pulling sheets from beds. Example: As the heaviest of several job duties, worker lifts, pushes, and pulls to jack an automobile, remove tire from wheel, and remount tire on wheel.

Heavy Work: Lifting 100 lb maximum with frequent lifting or carrying objects that weigh up to 50 lb. Example: Worker pushes handtrucks up and down aisles of warehouse to fill orders, stoops to lift cartons of items with an average weight of 65 lb, and places them on the truck. Example: Worker digs a trench by hand to specified depth and width using a shovel.

VII. Physical Barriers

	Yes	No
PARKING		
1. Is parking provided that is adjacent or convenient to building?	___	___
2. Is route from parking to building barrier free?	___	___
3. Is space indicated for handicapped?	___	___
4. Is space at least 12 feet wide?	___	___
RAMP		
5. Is ramp available for access to building?	___	___
6. Is ramp at least 45 inches wide?	___	___
7. Is slope no more than 1 inch in rise to 12 inches in length?	___	___
8. Does ramp have at least one handrail?	___	___
9. Does ramp have landings at top and bottom for 5 inches in direction of travel?	___	___
BUILDING ENTRANCE		
10. Is at least one accessible building entrance a main entrance?	___	___
11. Does door require less than 8 lb of force to open?	___	___
12. Is there a minimum 32-inch clearance?	___	___
13. In direction of door swing, is there an area at least 5 inches by 5 feet?	___	___
14. Is the threshold flat or with a maximum 1/2-inch slope?	___	___
ELEVATORS		
15. Are elevators directly accessible from a usable entrance?	___	___
16. Is office or work site directly accessible from usable main entrance or from elevator?	___	___
17. Does elevator car automatically come within 1/2 inch of building floor?	___	___
18. Are the highest controls within 54 inches of the floor?	___	___
19. Do elevator panels have braille and raised arabic symbols to right of buttons?	___	___
FLOORS		
20. Are floors of a smooth, nonslip material or covered with low-nap carpet?	___	___

	Yes	No

DOORS
21. Do doors within work sites have a 32-inch clear opening? ____ ____
22. Are doors opened by lever handles rather than door knobs? ____ ____
23. Are thresholds sloped and less than 1/2 inch high? ____ ____
24. Are passageways at least 48 inches wide and free of tight turns? ____ ____
25. Can existing obstructions within passageways or office be easily moved? ____ ____

RESTROOM
26. Is restroom convenient and accessible to work site? ____ ____
27. Do entry doors have 32-inch clear opening? ____ ____
28. Is passageway from restroom entrance to stall 43 inches wide at all points? ____ ____
29. If there is a vestibule between two doors, is it at least 5-1/2 feet long? ____ ____
30. Is there at least 29 inches of vertical clearance under sink? ____ ____
31. Are the sink controls the single-lever type? ____ ____
32. Does at least one restroom stall have a 30-inch clear entrance? ____ ____
33. Does stall door open out? ____ ____
34. Is stall at least 36 inches wide? ____ ____
35. Is the distance from the front of the stool to the closed door at least 48 inches? ____ ____
36. Is there a grab bar on each side of stall? ____ ____
37. Are the grab bars parallel to and 33 inches from floor? ____ ____

WATER FOUNTAIN
38. Is one water fountain no more than 36 inches from floor, or has a cup dispenser been provided? ____ ____
39. Is there 27-inch knee clearance beneath fountain? ____ ____
40. Are spout and controls in front? ____ ____

TELEPHONE
41. Is telephone available and accessible for use? ____ ____
42. If not, is a public phone in an accessible area? ____ ____
43. Is one telephone mounted so that the highest operable parts are no more than 54 inches above the floor? ____ ____
44. Does the booth entrance provide 30-inch wide clearance? ____ ____

TRAVEL
45. Does job require travel to noncompany sites that may not be accessible? ____ ____

Source: Michelle Demore-Taber, M.S., CRC/LRC, licensed rehab. counselor.

Index